Suzette,
Thank you
for all the positive
thoughts for our
Austin! It takes
a village —
Love + hugs —
Karen

The Right Rehab

Praise for *The Right Rehab*

"A necessary and timely book dealing with a serious health issue that is mostly ignored. *The Right Rehab* is an easily understandable book about the serious issue of drug disease and how to deal with it. A must-read for anyone dealing with the drug dependency disease. As a father who lost a son to this disease, I wish the book had been available when it would have helped me most." —**Robert Shapiro, Esq.**, partner, Glaser Weil

"A must-read guide for anyone trying to make sense of the confusing world of addiction treatment, insurance coverage, and the various aspects of recovery. This is an important and relevant book that will not only educate but also, and most important, help save lives." —**Michael Neatherton**, CEO, Solution Point; former chairman, Northbound Treatment Services; former COO, Betty Ford Center

"An amazing resource for every family. From intervention to sustained recovery, Walter Wolf has provided a 'what you need to know' road map to navigate your way down the addiction treatment highway." —**Mike Early**, forty-year treatment executive formerly with Northbound Treatment Services; Caron Foundation; Hazelden Foundation

"*The Right Rehab* shows families how to learn the strategies for coping with an addicted family member, ensure their resources are well spent and effective over the long term, and begin the process of repairing the very real PTSD that can come from the chaos of addiction and serious mental illness." —**Kevin McCauley**, MD, senior fellow, The Meadows of Wickenburg

"This is a remarkable book and irreplaceable resource for any family dealing with substance use and mental health crises. Wolf has produced the most effective, cogent, comprehensive, and clear how-to-guide for helping a loved one in need. In my experience as a lawyer with decades of sobriety, working in the field of lawyer recovery and wellness, *The Right Rehab* is the single best available guide to what we need to know about treatment options and recovery. I personally recommend that anyone who faces family substance use issues get this book and become familiar with it. It will save lives." —**Dan McDermott**, executive director, Florida Lawyers Assistance, Inc.

"*The Right Rehab* is every family's frame of reference when searching for a loved one's addiction treatment. It is invaluable." —**Chico West**, founder and owner, Casa Colina Addiction Treatment Center

"What a tremendous resource for not only those suffering from alcoholism and addiction but also, and just as important, their friends and family. The detail in this book is impeccable. It is such a well-written, comprehensive guide that helps one navigate the early questions of 'What do we do?' through all of the twists and turns, until those afflicted with this disease are in sustained, life-long recovery. Wolf is tremendous—God bless him!" —**Michael A. McCormick**, DO, medical director, Health Care Professionals Unit, Caron Treatment Centers

"Finding the right treatment for you or your loved one can be the difference between success and failure or, in many cases, life and death. Wolf knows this field and, through *The Right Rehab*, brilliantly navigates the complicated labyrinth of addiction treatment." —**Jeffrey Klein**, executive director, Crownview Co-Occurring Institute

"A real strength of this book is its ability to take complex, daunting situations and break them down into more understandable and manageable elements. The combination of practical information and concrete, straightforward steps should provide a valuable resource in helping families and loved ones impacted by addiction obtain the assistance so desperately needed." —**Gregory L. Futral, PhD**, Pine Grove Behavioral Health and Addiction Services

"As a criminal defense attorney, I have many clients in desperate need of drug rehabilitation and mental health intervention. Mr. Wolf has helped guide me, my clients, and their families to and through the right places for each person's very particular situation. He not only knows what facilities are available across the nation but also knows how to interface with them and how to navigate the insurance maze. He is a true expert. This book serves as an excellent guide to anyone dealing with these issues." —**Laura K. Deskin**, attorney at law, Oklahoma City, Oklahoma

"Required reading for those who come face-to-face with addiction of a loved one. Told with crystal clarity, *The Right Rehab* gives expert advice on addiction recovery from therapeutic choices to payment options. It is a wealth of knowledge." —**Stanley Hupfeld**, former CEO of Integris Health of Oklahoma

"*The Right Rehab* should be required reading for every parent when their loved one needs treatment for substance use and/or mental disorder." —**Heath Chitwood**, executive director, Still Waters

"Based on his very own personal experience, Wolf composed this amazing step-by-step guide on how to be prepared to make pivotal decisions if substance abuse strikes your family. A must-read for every afflicted family desperately trying to save a loved one." —**Britta K. Ostermeyer**, MD, MBA, DFAPA, Paul and Ruth Jonas Chair in Mental Health, professor and chairman, University of Oklahoma Health Sciences Center

"Masterful! Wolf outlines vital information families must know and critical steps families must take to ensure that they are making an informed decision about treatment for a loved one. Recovery is a very real possibility with the correct diagnosis and a treatment plan that is individualized, integrated, and intentional." —**Julio I. Rojas, PhD**, associate professor of psychiatry and behavioral sciences, University of Oklahoma College of Medicine

"Wolf has written an explicit and thorough guide through the labyrinth that is modern drug and alcohol treatment in America. Anyone seeking help for a friend or family member suffering from the disease of addiction should read this book." —**John Hiatt**, nine-time Grammy Award–nominated singer/songwriter

"For over twenty-five years, I have witnessed families and clients in crisis scurry to find the best treatment option. Many are very uninformed and desperately trying to learn all they can within a twenty-four-hour period! Mr. Wolf succinctly details what should be considered when seeking help. There is not a 'one size fits all' treatment center; every client needs to have a treatment experience that best fits their specific needs. Thank you, Mr. Wolf, for writing a comprehensive, easy-to-understand resource to assist those in need. This book is a beautiful guide and a true gift." —**Christi Cessna**, MS, CEO, Integrative Life Network

"In the past three decades, addiction treatment and recovery have become a big industry. Anytime an industry experiences rapid growth, the field can range from intelligent and thoughtful care to charlatans and creeps out to make the fastest buck. Wolf's book, inspired by his desire to care for a family member, is a practical and concise guide to finding the proper treatment for family members facing the heartbreaking crisis of addiction." —**Jeff Greenberg**, CEO, Village Studios

Sample of Client Testimonials

"Walter Wolf personally knows the places and programs because he has personal, family experience with the same problems. He is that rare professional who cares." —**G. H.**, Nashville, Tennessee

"Calling Walter was one of the best decisions I've ever made—he knows what needs to be done. Now we have recovery, hope, peace, and continued support from Walter. He saved our lives." —**Diane W.**, Edmond, Oklahoma

"Not only did his referrals to rehabilitation facilities and a criminal defense attorney prove invaluable, but Walter's genuine concern and unwavering support assured us that we were not alone during those dark days. We consider ourselves extremely lucky to have crossed paths with Walter Wolf— our heartfelt thanks!" —**David F.**, Richmond, Virginia

"Due to his intervention and relationships with the best treatment facilities in the country, Walter has the experience necessary to navigate the world of insurance and negotiating payment plans. Thanks to Walter, our son and family are whole again." —**Beth and Ron D.**, Seattle, Washington

"When you live with an addict, you live in constant chaos. When my family member finally reached out for help, Walter was such a solid resource as to what was best for our situation—financially, emotionally, and psychologically." —**Elaine H.**, Denver, Colorado

"Walter made it possible for me to create a strong foundation for my recovery. Presently, I am four years, four months, three weeks, and three days clean and sober with a happy and full life. Thank you, Walter, for helping me find my own solutions." —**Steven W.**, Eugene, Oregon

"I vividly remember the day I called my mom in tears. All I could say was 'I need help.' The two different treatment centers where I was sent had different evaluations, and neither could help me. It wasn't until my family was put in contact with Walter that my life began to change. He knew what to do. He found a rehab that was right for me and my family through every stage of the process. Today, I am almost three years sober and finally have a life worth living. I have finished my bachelor's degree, have begun building a career as a legal assistant, help other women in recovery, and now have loving, honest relationships with my friends and family. Most important, I now love myself and the life I am building. Without Walter, I would not be who I am today." —**Kay L.**, Newport Beach, California

The Right Rehab

A Guide to Addiction and Mental Illness Recovery When Crisis Hits Your Family

Walter Wolf

Rowman & Littlefield
Lanham • Boulder • New York • London

Published by Rowman & Littlefield
An imprint of The Rowman & Littlefield Publishing Group, Inc.
4501 Forbes Boulevard, Suite 200, Lanham, Maryland 20706
www.rowman.com

86-90 Paul Street, London EC2A 4NE, United Kingdom

Illustrations by Todd Pendleton

British Library Cataloguing in Publication Information Available

Library of Congress Cataloging-in-Publication Data

Names: Wolf, Walter, 1953– author.
Title: The right rehab : a guide to addiction and mental illness recovery when crisis hits your family / Walter Wolf.
Description: Lanham : Rowman & Littlefield, [2021] | Includes bibliographical references and index. | Summary: "Those with substance abuse issues often have family and friends who wish to help, but knowing how to find and access the right rehab for a loved one can be confusing, costly, and even inappropriate in some cases. Here, Walter Wolf guides readers through the process from crisis to placement to recovery"— Provided by publisher.
Identifiers: LCCN 2021020011 (print) | LCCN 2021020012 (ebook) | ISBN 9781538155127 (cloth ; alk. paper) | ISBN 9781538155134 (epub)
Subjects: LCSH: Substance abuse—Treatment. | Substance abuse treatment facilities. | Addicts—Rehabilitation. | Mentally ill—Care.
Classification: LCC RC564 .W65 2021 (print) | LCC RC564 (ebook) | DDC 362.29—dc23
LC record available at https://lccn.loc.gov/2021020011
LC ebook record available at https://lccn.loc.gov/2021020012

♾️™ The paper used in this publication meets the minimum requirements of American National Standard for Information Sciences—Permanence of Paper for Printed Library Materials, ANSI/NISO Z39.48-1992.

"Until you've walked in the shoes of somebody who needs these substances, you can't possibly understand the tremendous gravitational pull of the compulsion to use." —Christopher Kennedy Lawford[1]

Several years ago, my lifelong friend Chris Lawford and I were reminiscing about our childhood and what we would change if given the chance. I made the wisecrack that he obviously would choose not being an addict for nine years of his life. Chris said, "No, I wouldn't change a thing." What? Who in their right mind would choose to be a heroin addict if given the chance to go back in time and change that? He explained that if not for that life, "I wouldn't be the person I am today."

His life of knowledge, experience, friendships, and a deep, deep appreciation for his spiritual life never would have happened if not for his addiction. Most of all, he was there for me and my family as well as the endless number of souls struggling with the same affliction. Chris's recovery saved not only his own life but also the lives of countless others.

Chris's addiction and recovery also brought me an unexpected gift. If not for them, I would not have the tools, relationships, and resources I have today to help make families whole again; I also would not have written this book.

Tragically, we unexpectedly lost Chris in 2018. Due to his addiction, he repeatedly said he knew the years he was living were a gift, and when the time came, his goal was to die sober.

Chris achieved that goal, although way too soon.

Bless you, Christopher.

---

1. Christopher Kennedy Lawford, *Recover to Live: Kick Any Habit, Manage Any Addiction* (Dallas, TX: BenBella Books, 2013), 38.

CONTENTS

ACKNOWLEDGMENTS

I cannot do justice to the help and support I received in making this book possible. But for my professional responsibility of confidentiality, they know who they are, and I have acknowledged that personally to each and every one of them.

Those whom I can mention are my attorney, Peter Dekom, and agents, Joel Gotler and Murray Weiss. Their guidance, judgment, and encouragement have been indispensable.

Suzanne Staszak-Silva, my editor at Rowman & Littlefield, is the reason why this book is a published work. Without hers and her assistant Deni Remsberg's belief and dedication, a countless number of terrified families would still be prey for unscrupulous grifters and con artists. I wish to thank you and your colleagues at Rowman & Littlefield for your patience and belief in me.

Rob Jolles coached me in how to go from idea to written word. I cannot thank him enough for his leadership, experience, and confidence in me. Rob, I hope you are proud.

The researchers at the Substance Abuse and Mental Health Services Administration (SAMHSA) are the unsung heroes of the professionals who have dedicated their lives to the treatment of addiction and mental illness. Their thorough, exhaustive, and encyclopedic research is a shining example of our tax dollars at work for the betterment of humanity. Thank you.

Finally, enough cannot be said for the treatment professionals throughout our nation. It takes a special type of person to go to work each day knowing that there's a good chance their work will meet with failure. But relapse is frequently part of the journey, and it's the patients who eventually succeed, who attain a life of recovery, who drive those health care professionals to keep striving to change people's lives. Those professionals save families. They are loved. When you meet one, thank them for what they do. They are on the side of the angels.

INTRODUCTION

You are reading this for any number of reasons . . .

You got a call in the middle of the night announcing that a loved one is in the hospital due to a drug overdose, an accident due to alcohol or illicit drug use, or a violent incident related to drug use—or she's in the psych unit due to a psychotic break induced by substance use or a mental disorder.

Perhaps the call is from the police department because your loved one is in jail for a DUI or a felony related to illicit drugs.

Or, like millions of families throughout our nation, you have a family member suffering from SUD (substance use disorder), and, despite your desperate pleas to get help, nothing has changed—until now. You've finally had enough.

It could be that you know a family (most of us do) going through any number of the previous scenarios and they need help.

If you're a parent, nothing stirs your fear and emotions more than when your child is controlled by drugs or alcohol. How do I know this? Because ten years ago I got that call, the call that my child was in crisis due to addiction—an addiction my wife and I had no idea existed.

All these scenarios have one thing in common: you're totally lost. You're asking yourself, "What the hell do I know about addiction, about rehab? Who can tell me what I need to know—right now?"

Although I didn't know anything about addiction, I knew who did. One of my closest friends was a high-profile member of the recovery community. All he had to do was make one phone call. Within twenty-four hours, my loved one was in detox at one of the finest rehabs on the planet.

I was lucky, but I couldn't help but think about those who aren't as lucky, those without trusted connections into the treatment world. What do they do? How do they know who to call and who to trust? How do they know which rehab actually delivers what it promises without ripping off their hard-earned money? But most of all, how do they treat their loved one?

That middle-of-the-night phone call did more than change my family; it made me who I am today—an interventionist working with families across the nation in finding the right treatment options when addiction and/or mental disorder hits them.

Addiction attacks families at every socioeconomic level—from Park Avenue to Skid Row. Its victims are parents, mothers, fathers, children, brothers, sisters, grandchildren, aunts, uncles, friends— and yourself. It doesn't matter whether one is male or female, employed or unemployed, young or old, any race or religion: everyone is fair game. Many don't appear to have addiction issues at all. In fact, many of those who are dependent on drugs or alcohol are "functional." They have jobs and live with their families, but the disease will worsen over time. Seventy-five percent of those with SUD are actively employed—55 percent of them full-time.[1]

The call for help, no matter who it's from, is the precise time when families are the most vulnerable, desperate to find the right treatment solution. If you are successful in getting your loved one into treatment, there will be not only dark days but also days of hope and progress. During your journey, you'll most likely learn six key lessons.

First, addiction is a family disease. Although one person is addicted, it affects the entire family. With more than sixteen thousand treatment facilities across our nation, how could the uninitiated possibly know which is the right one for their family member or oneself? I've received countless calls from families for help. Those appeals made me realize that this book is one whose time has come when addiction or mental illness hits your family.

Second, addiction is a chronic brain disease resulting in the inability to control the impulse to use a substance or stop repeating a process despite devastating consequences. It is not the result of a moral failing, bad character, or lack of will, though some unenlightened people still believe that. It is a chronic disease that alters a person's brain structure and function; it cannot be stopped by a simple "Just say no" or "Buck up, will ya!"

Third, a mental disorder more often than not accompanies addiction. The question is which one is driving the other. I am not a psychologist, therapist, or drug treatment counselor with degrees/qualifications after my name, but I know enough to know that all diagnoses and treatment must emanate from licensed, certified, experienced, and caring professionals. Period.

Fourth, I learned from those in recovery that the resources don't get the victim sober. They are only the tools helping the individual get sober. Sobriety occurs when the victim genuinely wants to get sober and is willing to put in the work to get there—it is completely up to the individual. Most important, those in recovery can live full, productive, meaningful, significant lives just like everyone else who has never suffered from addiction.

Fifth, in my experience, relapse is often part of the journey (especially for millennials), not the failure of treatment. I've seen families lament, "Well, there goes that money down the drain . . . what good did that rehab do when she goes back to using drugs?" It's a hard and expensive lesson, but nonetheless one to learn. More than 60 percent of those treated for SUD relapse within the first year of discharge from treatment—similar to relapse rates of other chronic diseases such as diabetes, hypertension, and asthma. That's when it's time to reinstate treatment, albeit with adjustments (or even a completely different approach). Even after a year or two of remission achieved through treatment and aftercare, it can take three to five more years before the risk of relapse drops below 15 percent (the level of risk that people in the general population have of developing an SUD in their lifetime).[2]

Sixth, there is no such thing as "the best rehab." It doesn't exist. What does exist is the *right* rehab for a particular individual. Lists of the "100 best rehabs" are a marketing and advertising ploy. Don't fall for it. The "best" rehab is the *right* rehab that best matches an individual's diagnosis; substance use patterns; related medical, mental, and social issues; and resources—to mention a few crucial factors. When it comes to treatment facilities, one size does *not* fit all.

Lifeboat

In 1944, Alfred Hitchcock directed the two-time Oscar-winning film *Lifeboat*, starring Tallulah Bankhead. Taking place in a lifeboat of survivors from a ship torpedoed by a U-boat during World War II, the film depicts a diverse group of strangers brought together by chance who now depend on each other to survive under the grimmest of circumstances.

Throughout the drama, each character's wants, fears, and dreams are slowly revealed in what turns out to be a prolonged group therapy session punctuated by intermittent bouts of panic and heroism. By the end of the film, they are saved by their ingenuity, but mostly because they had no other choice but to trust each other if they were to survive. Strangers at first, they now forever share an unbreakable bond of wisdom and trust forged through their shared experience of horror and survival.

That classic black-and-white movie is a perfect metaphor for family group therapy during family week at a treatment facility or at an Al-Anon meeting. They are thrown together as strangers—young, old, wealthy, poor, native-born, immigrants, Black, white,

Asian, Latino—who under any other circumstances would never cross each other's paths, let alone confess their innermost fears, flaws, and inadequacies *to complete strangers* but for this plague of addiction. You arrive as strangers but leave as brothers and sisters, knowing that you and your family are *not* the only ones clawing through the gauntlet of your loved one's addiction. Your fears, regrets, and love for your afflicted family member are validated by new allies in your collective struggle to save your family.

Likewise, think of this book as a lifeboat helping you and your family survive in that churning sea of treatment charlatans, impostors, and opportunists who are circling for a feeding frenzy on families like yours at your most vulnerable time. At $42 billion per year[3] and growing, drug and alcohol treatment is an unregulated industry creating millionaires out of unscrupulous owners of testing, online marketing, and treatment centers.

This book is for the more than sixty-one million Americans and their families suffering from SUD and/or a mental disorder. That's the populations of California, Oregon, Washington, Idaho, Montana, and Nevada combined. If you're reading this book because you are in the same situation, the first thing to know is that you are not alone. Nearly one-third of our nation's families are impacted by addiction. It's nearly impossible to speak with someone who's not dealing with addiction and/or mental illness in their family or at least knows of a family who is.

As a survivor, my role now is to use my unique resources, relationships, and experience to help other families on their journey through intervention and providing the treatment options available according to their resources.

> "Today we have so many treatment centers popping up across the country, trying out new strategies and protocols that will differentiate them from the pack, but that aren't necessarily effective. This makes it difficult for families to evaluate treatment options. It's difficult to be smart consumers in a confusing arena."
>
> —Debra Jay[4]

Since this book did not exist when I needed it, I decided to write it myself.

At the beginning of my family's crisis, I stood at the foot of the Mount Everest of learning curves. The purpose of this book is to dramatically shorten that learning curve for families in the same in-crisis situation. It was then that I realized there has to be a dedicated, objective source helping families learn about the honest, ethical, trustworthy, evidence-based options available for those who are about to enter a world fraught with those who will do them harm. But it is also a world with those who know their pain and are there to guide them and their family to a life of recovery.

The title of this book is *The Right Rehab* because you are trying to save a loved one who's in crisis. The last thing you want to do is read a book, but you need to know how to get the right care. As my friends in South Africa say—you need it NOW-NOW!

That's why chapters 1–6 are summarized like a step-by-step user guide with the information you need to know immediately—like where I was at the beginning of my "what the hell do I do now?" journey. Chapter 7, "Cheat Sheet: A Summary of What You Need to Know Now-Now," is a compilation of summaries of those preceding six chapters, making it easy for the reader to go directly to them without even having to read the chapters—or, at the very least, the chapter summaries serve as easy reference material.

Also, you'll notice that when referring to the one suffering from addiction, I don't use the term *addict*. Too frequently it is used as a pejorative and disparaging label. It is not the correct way to refer to someone suffering from the *disease* of addiction. Would you describe a cancer patient or one fighting diabetes using a term that connotes a lack of character or low morals—as if they got what they deserved? Addiction is a chronic brain disease, not a result of weakened willpower or a lack of morals. Like those with other life-threatening diseases, those battling addiction are "victims" or "patients," and they deserve the same respect.

I have tried my best to use gender-neutral language, but when necessary to describe a nonspecific individual, I will alternate between she/her and he/him throughout the book.

I like to think of *The Right Rehab* as a user guide for families who find themselves navigating the difficult road of addiction and/or mental illness. I hope you think of it that way as well.

Godspeed,
Walter Wolf

BREAKING THE GLASS

Do This Now

If you are reading this because you or your family are in crisis due to drug/alcohol addiction and/or mental illness, you are likely experiencing a thousand nightmares right now. Your first priority is getting the victim to a safe place, ensuring his immediate health and well-being, and then getting you and your family stabilized.

Immediately call 911 if the individual is suffering from an apparent overdose or a psychotic break, or if she is threatening to harm herself or anyone else. Ask for an officer trained in crisis intervention to accompany the responders.

Immediately call 911 if the person is unconscious. If you suspect a drug overdose, apply Narcan if available. Narcan is today's fire extinguisher. If you have a family or household member you either know or suspect of being a substance user, it would be prescient to have multiple doses of Narcan within easy reach. When you consider that "over 81,000 deaths occurred in the United States in the 12 months ending in May 2020,"[1] this precaution could easily save your loved one. Be ready to apply CPR if the person is not breathing or doesn't have a pulse.

If the individual is in acute withdrawal (negative emotions, pain, sweating, intestinal distress, intense craving, seizures[2]), call 911. You could also take him yourself to your local ER, crisis intervention center, or detox center if the symptoms are not yet acute.

If your loved one is under arrest or in jail and you know or have access to a criminal defense attorney, call them. The attorney can find out easier than you about any outstanding warrants, whether the jail already processed the person, and whether bail has been set.

Have This Ready

During this crisis, you will be asked for specific information about the individual. The more accessible the information, the smoother and more efficient the process will be. The sooner you have this information together, the sooner you can get your loved one on the road to recovery.

Personal

- Age and birthdate
- Address of residence
- Names, phone numbers, and relationship of essential contacts
- Social Security number
- Spouse or significant other's addiction status
- Number of dependents
- Current service member or veteran status
- Employment status
- Insurance status

Per the Health Insurance Portability and Accountability Act (HIPPA) laws, determine who should have consent to speak with the facility and know the patient's medical situation.

Substance Abuse

- What is the individual's drug(s) of choice?
- How often and for how long has the person been using?

- Does the individual deny there's a problem?
- How many other instances of crisis or emergencies have occurred?
- Has the individual undergone previous treatment for SUDs and/or mental illness?
- Does the person use at home or away?
- Does the individual habitually disappear for long periods?
- Is there a current or past diagnosis?
- Does the individual admit substance use?
- Is the person willing to go to treatment?
- From where and from whom does the individual acquire substances?
- How does the person have the resources to pay for the substances?

Individual and Family Medical History

- What is the individual's history of substance abuse and/or mental illness?
- What is the family history regarding substance abuse and/or mental illness?
- Has the individual been diagnosed by a health care professional?
- Does a family member have access to the individual's medical records?
- Are medical records available?
- Does the individual have a primary
  - physician? If so, provide contact information.
  - therapist? If so, provide contact information.
  - counselor? If so, provide contact information.
- Is the person currently being treated for any malady?
- What medications are prescribed to the individual currently?
- Where are the medications?
- Is the individual a danger to self or others?

- Is there a history of suicide ideation?
- Has the individual ever suffered from a traumatic brain injury (TBI)?
- Is there a history of trauma or posttraumatic stress disorder (PTSD)?
- Does the individual live alone or with others?
- What is the status of the individual's relationship with other family members?

Legal

- Does the individual have a guardian or someone with a power of attorney (POA)?
- Is there an existing will?
- Is there a living will?
- Is there a "do not resuscitate" (DNR) order in place?
- Is there a history of convictions, incarceration, arrests, or DUIs?
- Is the individual currently on parole or probation?
- Are there any outstanding warrants?
- Has the person participated in drug court?
- Are there any upcoming court dates?
- Does the individual have criminal defense attorney? If so, provide contact information.
- Is the person in need of an attorney?
- Is the individual under the supervision of a probation or parole officer? If so, provide contact information.

When You Need a Lawyer

If criminal justice is a player in this scenario, you'll need a criminal defense attorney. If money is an issue—it usually is—don't ask Uncle Bob who practices real estate law to represent your loved one for free. Instead, ask Bob to recommend a defense lawyer. And don't be afraid of going to the Mt. Olympus of firms in your area to ask for representation even if you think there's no way you could afford them. You never know unless you ask! Firms take on cases for all kinds of reasons. Yours may be one of them. Go for it.

Also, don't be shy in asking the attorney about a payment plan to satisfy the fee. You'd be surprised how many of them accommodate their clients that way. If they are unable to fit your resources, ask them for recommendations—they will know who is right for your situation. Plus, calling an attorney saying that someone from a big-shot law firm referred you could be advantageous for both of you.

There is also the public defender's office. It's natural for people to attach little to no value to a service they get for free. In my experience, if given the choice between a seasoned public defender (PD) and a relatively young and inexperienced attorney at a private law firm, I'll take the PD any day. Being a PD means jumping into the fire immediately upon joining the team, which translates into experience—vastly more than a young associate at a firm.

When I started my practice, one defense attorney who represented several of my clients was, at forty-one years old, running his own practice and already one of the state's top lawyers. I asked why he had even bothered starting his career in the PD's office when he clearly would have been a star at a white-shoe firm.

"Walter," he said, "if I had started my career at a firm, it would have taken several years to be the lead lawyer on a murder case. When you work in the PD's office, you start immediately. Where else can you gain such a vast amount of experience in such a short amount of time?" Plus, in working daily with the key players of that county's criminal justice system—prosecutors, judges, clerks of the court, bailiffs, secretaries in the DA's office, jailors, police officers, bondsmen—a young attorney quickly acquires knowledge and relationships that turn out to be invaluable to their clients.

Questions you should ask if your loved one is dealing with the criminal justice system include the following: Is this the defendant's first arrest? Have charges been filed? Has an arraignment date been set? Which judge has been appointed? Has bond been set? Could the person be released on OR (own recognizance), or will you need a bail bondsman? Should you even bail the person out? Keeping your loved one incarcerated for the short term will keep her from overdosing or getting into more legal trouble. At least you'll know where your loved one is.

When Treatment Is the Next Stage

Does the person want to go to treatment, or is he in denial about having a substance use and/or mental disorder? It's remarkable to see a defendant who is resistant to treatment all of a sudden be a convert when given the choice of going to treatment now or taking his chances with a trial and jail or prison later. If criminal justice is not in the picture and the individual is in denial about a problem or resistant to treatment, staging an intervention involving friends, family, and interested parties cutting off the enablement that allows the individual to continue his or her destructive behavior is most likely the next step.

Whether or not criminal justice issues are in the picture, and assuming treatment is the next stage, is there a diagnosis by a trained, certified health care professional of substance abuse or a mental disorder? Substance abuse *and* a mental disorder? If both, that means dual-diagnosis or co-occurring disorders. In that case, an experienced practitioner must determine which is the primary and which the secondary disorder.

Out of the more than sixteen thousand treatment programs and facilities in our nation, how do you know which program is the right one? Which ones actually deliver what they promise? How do you avoid being duped? How much can you afford to pay, even with insurance? What if you cannot pay? Are there still treatment programs available to you? How long should the treatment program last? Thirty, sixty, ninety, or 120 days? Six months? One year? Should the facility be local or out of state?

These are just a few of the issues you will be confronting. You've gotten this far. The following pages are designed to help guide you through the next stages of this terrifying, emotionally draining process.

WHAT IS TREATMENT?

"Your loved one is not at fault for having a disease, but he or she is responsible for getting treatment."[1]

"The goal of treatment is remission leading to lasting recovery."[2]

What Causes Addiction?

Several experts believe that addiction is a chronic, long-term illness resulting from the complex interplay between a person's genes and environment. Factors that are believed to contribute to an individual's addiction include the following:

- Physical, emotional, or sexual abuse and/or trauma (you don't have to be an Afghanistan or Iraq veteran to be suffering from posttraumatic stress disorder [PTSD])
- Neglect
- Family history of addiction
- Parental substance use
- Family and peer dynamics
- Household instability
- Availability of drugs or alcohol
- Exposure to stress

- Incarceration of family members
- Poverty
- Age when use begins
- Presence of a co-occurring mental disorder
- Little to no access to social support

Renowned addiction specialist Dr. Kevin McCauley adds the following insights:

"Addiction is a disorder of pleasure": He says, "At its heart, addiction is a disorder in the brain's ability to properly perceive pleasure. In the same way that blind people cannot perceive light, or a deaf person cannot perceive sound, addicts cannot perceive pleasure correctly—and that undermines their ability to make choices."

"Addiction is a disorder of choice": He continues, "Our capacity for free will, volition [act of choosing], agency . . . rests upon proper processing deeper in the brain. You have to have a perfectly functioning reward system that has to be firing on all 12 cylinders if we're going to make decisions that are really considerate of past consequences and future consequences and in line with our values."

"Addiction is caused by stress": Finally, he says, "What's at the core of the reward system is the chemical dopamine . . . and it turns out that [a] defect in the dopamine system can be caused by all different types of stress, especially early stress—early, continuous, poorly managed, even inherited stress can affect the functioning of the dopamine system."[3]

However, as with other chronic diseases like hypertension, asthma, or diabetes, there is no "cure," though it is manageable. Addiction can be managed so that anyone in recovery can live a self-directed, full, active, meaningful, loving, and productive life just like anyone else can do on this planet.

> "Addiction is a chronic brain disease, that has the potential for both recurrence (relapse) and recovery."
>
> —Vivek H. Murthy (MD, MBA),
> U.S. surgeon general, 2014–2017, 2021–[4]

Physical Dependence

Many people mistake physical dependence as addiction. It's not. Physical dependence accompanies addiction when the body adapts to the physical effects of a substance. Addiction, however, is characterized by an inability to stop using a substance resulting in devastating consequences such as failure to meet work, social, or family obligations—and, of course, death. The person's life revolves around getting that substance. For instance, I have a physical dependence on caffeine, but I don't have to spend my life constantly near a Starbucks, nor do I go on a crusade to find coffee if I don't have any at home. Quit coffee and endure two weeks of headaches—no biggie. Addiction—that's a different story.

After I had spinal surgery recently, the post-op pain really, really sucked. I used oxycodone with acetaminophen for eight days before switching to ibuprofen. I spent the next two miserable, restless nights unable to stay in one position long enough to fall asleep. I realized my body was dependent upon oxycodone's effect after only eight days of its use! Fortunately, my physical dependence didn't evolve into "I gotta have it or else," but I learned how it could have taken over my life. That's scary stuff when you realize that 168 million opioid prescriptions were written in 2019. That's a rate of 51.4 prescriptions per every one hundred American adults—and that's down from a record 81.3 per one hundred American adults in 2012. That is crazy![5]

Addiction/Substance Use Disorder (SUD) Treatment

> "Today, my best advice to people who are facing those difficult days of sobriety is to get humble. Make recovery your absolute priority over everything else."
>
> —Elton John[6]

Treatment. We hear that word constantly, but how many really know what it means when it comes to addiction and/or mental disorders? A common misconception about treatment is likening it to going to the emergency room to stitch up an injury. A few weeks later and presto, no more stitches—you're fixed, and you rarely think about them again.

Unlike stitches, addiction, like mental illness, is always with you. As chronic illnesses, they never go away, but you can learn to manage them so they don't manage you.

Treatment is not a cure, but it enables people to counteract addiction's disruptive effects on their brain and behavior to regain control of their lives.[7]

The key component of treatment is evidence-based therapy, which is combined with medication and recovery support services (RSS). RSS is intended as a continuum of care and lifestyle intended to support long-term recovery. How long does that take? "A lifetime" is what my friends in recovery tell me.

The brain is made up of brain cells—eighty-six billion of them. That's a big playing field, so the lifelong changes that need to take place understandably take time. My friends living in long-term recovery say that it's after five years of sobriety when they can confidently say they are in recovery, but they still live "one day at a time." Even after a year or two of remission is achieved—through treatment or some other route—it can take four to five more years before the risk of relapse drops below 15 percent, the level of risk that people in the general population have of developing an SUD in their lifetime.[8]

Diagnosis

"It is during the treatment process that we begin to fully grasp the potent nature of what ails us. We start to prepare for what's next, the rest of our lives."

—William Cope Moyers[9]

The professionals I know who work in the recovery sector emphasize that the same treatment is not right for every person or the accompanying disorder. To have the optimum chance of success, treatment professionals say the outcome depends on a few core factors:

- The extent and nature of the individual's problems
- The appropriateness of the formal treatment
- Ongoing services and mutual-aid support after formal treatment
- The level of honesty and bond shared among the individual, others in recovery, and the care providers
- The patient's age, gender, ethnicity, culture, and economic status
- The individual's trauma history
- Most of all, the patient's motivation to get and remain sober

In order to treat SUD, it is necessary to know exactly what needs to be treated, so let's start with the nature of an individual's problems. It's not enough to observe that "so and so has a drinking problem and needs to go to rehab." Says who? How serious is it? What needs to be treated? Is there something else going on—a co-occurring disorder such as PTSD, depression, anxiety, bipolar disorder? Is alcohol the only substance being abused? Is the individual in denial, or does she want to get help? This is where the medical and mental health professionals need to step in.

The true diagnosis of SUD is principally based on a clinical assessment by a trained professional. A tool professionals use as a guide in formulating that judgment is the fifth edition of the *Diagnostic and Statistical Manual of Mental Disorders* (DSM-5). The DSM-5 lists eleven diagnostic symptoms that define whether there is a disorder and, if so, its severity:

- Using in larger amounts or for longer than intended
- Wanting to cut down or stop using, but not managing to do it
- Spending a lot of time to get, use, or recover from use

- Craving for the substance
- Inability to manage commitments due to use
- Continuing to use, even when it causes problems in relationships
- Giving up important activities because of use
- Continuing to use, even when it puts the user in danger
- Continuing to use, even when physical or psychological problems may be made worse by use
- Increasing tolerance to the substance
- Withdrawal symptoms

The DSM-5 defines the scale of severity under these parameters:

- Fewer than two symptoms = no disorder
- Two to three symptoms = mild disorder
- Four to five symptoms = moderate disorder
- Six or more symptoms = severe disorder

The Substance Abuse and Mental Health Services Administration (SAMHSA), an agency of the U.S. Department of Health and Human Services, states that 40–60 percent of all those suffering from a substance use disorder also have an accompanying mental disorder—called a "co-occurring disorder" or a "dual diagnosis." The most common disorders co-occurring with substance use range from depression, anxiety, bipolar disorder, schizophrenia, and PTSD. Eighty percent of my clients have been diagnosed as having co-occurring disorders, necessitating a treatment facility that knows how to treat both disorders concurrently.

A professional diagnosis normally comes up as one of the following:

- Substance use disorder (SUD)
- Mental disorder

- Primary SUD and secondary mental disorder
- Primary mental disorder and secondary SUD

In lieu of an upfront, in-person diagnosis—frequently due to a criminal justice issue or if the individual is in denial and uncooperative—an over-the-phone assessment of the individual by a facility is often the starting point for treatment. In those cases, the integrity of the facility doing the assessment is of vital importance.

Outpatient versus Inpatient

Outpatient treatment provides group and individual counseling in morning or evening sessions accommodating those who maintain a regular work or academic schedule. Typically, two kinds of treatment—intensive outpatient (IOP) and outpatient (OP)—are less expensive and intensive than residential treatment. Sessions are typically group programs at the initial level of care for those with mild to moderate SUDs or continuing care for those recently discharged from a residential program and live at home or in a sober living environment. Occasionally, the same clinics will also offer partial hospitalization programming (PHP), which is the more intensive all-day treatment.

Inpatient is a level of treatment easy to misinterpret. In drug treatment parlance, it refers to medically supervised substance withdrawal delivered in an acute, inpatient hospital or dedicated medical unit—otherwise known as *detox*. It also is a moniker for *residential care*—SUD treatment not in a hospital, but in a hospital-like setting that offers twenty-four-hour support, staff, and structure for intensive evidence-based clinical services and therapy. For those who are just out of detox, are prone to relapse, or have a co-occurring illness, residential treatment provides the twenty-four-hour care and support needed at that time.

For our purposes, inpatient detox is referred to as *detox* and inpatient residential as *residential*.

Addictions Treated

> "You know you're an alcoholic when you misplace things—like a decade."
>
> —Paul Williams[10]

Substance: A psychoactive compound with the potential to cause SUDs and other health and social problems.

Substance addiction: The most severe form of substance use, associated with compulsive or uncontrolled use of one or more substances.

Process addiction: Obsessive behavior not necessarily accompanied by substance use that compels the individual to engage compulsively and repeatedly in conduct detrimental to the individual.

Drug and alcohol treatment facilities treat addiction to substances that are primarily grouped into three major categories.

- Alcohol
  - Beer
  - Wine
  - Malt liquor
  - Distilled spirits
- Illicit drugs
  - Cocaine, including crack
  - Heroin
  - Hallucinogens: LSD, PCP, ecstasy, peyote, mescaline, psilocybin
  - Methamphetamines, including crystal meth
  - Marijuana, including hashish
  - Synthetic drugs: K2, spice, bath salts
  - Prescription-type medications
    - Pain relievers: synthetic, semi-synthetic, and non-synthetic opioid medications
      - Opium
      - Morphine
      - Fentanyl
      - Codeine

- • Oxycodone
- • Hydrocodone
- • Tramadol products
  - ■ Tranquilizers
    - • Benzodiazepines
    - • Meprobamate products
    - • Muscle relaxants
  - ■ Simulants and methamphetamine
    - • Amphetamine
    - • Dextroamphetamine
    - • Phentermine products
    - • Mazindol products
    - • Methylphenidate or dexmethylphenidate products
  - ■ Sedatives
    - • Temazepam
    - • Flurazepam
    - • Triazolam
    - • Any barbiturates
- • Over-the-counter drugs and other substances
  - ○ Cough and cold medicines
  - ○ Inhalants
    - ■ Amyl nitrite
    - ■ Cleaning fluids
    - ■ Gasoline
    - ■ Lighter gases
    - ■ Anesthetics
    - ■ Solvents
    - ■ Spray paint
    - ■ Nitrous oxide

I don't know about you, but I am easily confused when it comes to the pharmacological category of drugs sold as brand names that have become a common part of our lexicon. Hopefully, figures 2.1–2.4 will clarify the true nature of the drugs most of us legally (and perhaps sometimes illegally) ingest at some point in our lives.

Prescription
pain relievers

Hydrocodone Products

Vicodin®
Lortab®
Norco®
Zohydro® ER
Hydrocodone

Oxycodone Products

Oxycontin®
Percocet®
Percodan®
Roxicet®
Roxicodone®
Oxycodone

Tramadol Products

Ultram®
Ultram® ER
Ultracet®
Tramadol

Extended-Release
Tramadol

©The Right Rehab, LLC

Morphine Products

Avinza®
Kadian®
MS Contin®
Morphine

Extended-Release
Morphine

Fentanyl Products

Actiq®
Duragesic®
Fentora®
Fentanyl

Buprenorphine Products

Suboxone®
Buprenorphine

Oxymorphone Products

Opana®
Opanax® ER
Oxymorphone

Extended Release
Oxymorphone

Demoral®

Hydromorphone Products

Dilaudid® or
Hydromorphone
Exalgo® or
Extended-Release
Hydromorphone

Methadone

Other Prescription Pain Relievers

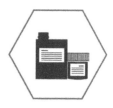

Figure 2.1.

Source: Substance Abuse and Mental Health Services Administration (2016, fig. 2). Art © The Right Rehab, LLC.

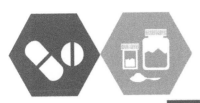

Prescription tranquilizers

Benzodiazepine Tranquilizers

Alprazolam Products

Xanax®
Xanax®XR
Alprazolam
Extended-Release Alprazoiam

Lorazepam Products

Ativan®
Lorazepam

Clonazepam Products

Klonopin®
Clonazepam

Diazepam Products

Valium®
Diazepam

Muscle Relaxants

Cyclobenzaprine (Also known as Flexeril®)

Soma®

Buspirone (Also known as BuSpar®)

Hydroxyzine (Also known as Atarax® or Vistaril®)

Meprobamate (Also known as Equanil® or Miltown®)

Other Prescription Tranquilizers

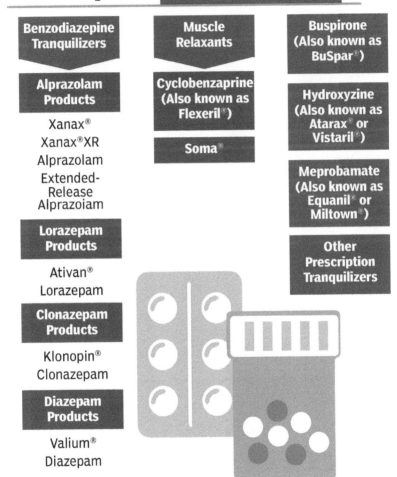

Figure 2.2.
Source: Substance Abuse and Mental Health Services Administration (2016, fig. 3). Art © The Right Rehab, LLC.

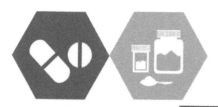

Prescription stimulants

Amphetamine Products	Methylphenidate Products	Anorectic (Weight Loss) Stimulants
Adderall®	Ritalin®	Didrex®
Adderall® XR	Ritalin® SR or LA	Benzphetamine
Dexedrine®	Concerta®	Tenuate®
Vyvanse®	Daytrana®	Diethylpropion
Dextroamphetamine	Metadate® CD	Phendimetrazine
	Metadate® ER	Phentermine
Amphetamine-Dextroamphetamine combinations	Focalin®	
	Focalin® XR	**Provigil®**
	Methylphenidate	
Extended Release Amphetamine-Dextroamphetamine Combinations	Extended Release Methylphenidate	**Other Prescription Stimulants**
	Dexmethylphenidate	
	Extended Release-Dexmethylphenidate	

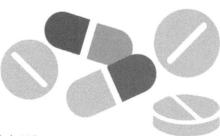

©The Right Rehab, LLC

Figure 2.3.

Source: Substance Abuse and Mental Health Services Administration (2016, fig. 4). Art © The Right Rehab, LLC.

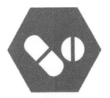

Prescription
sedatives

Zolpidem Products	Benzodiazepine Sedatives	Barbituates

Zolpidem Products

Ambien®

Ambien® CR

Zolpidem

Extended-Release Zolpidem

Eszopiclone Products

Lunesta® or Eszopiclone

Zaleplon Products

Sonata® or Zaleplon

Benzodiazepine Sedatives

Flurazepam (Also known as Dalmane®

Temazepam Products
|
Restoril®

Temazepam

Triazolam Products
|
Halcion

Triazolam

Barbituates

Butisol®

Seconal®

Phenobarbital

Other Prescription Sedatives

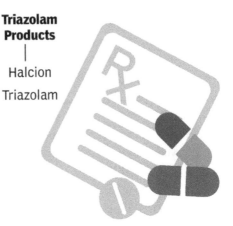

©The Right Rehab, LLC

Figure 2.4.

Source: Substance Abuse and Mental Health Services Administration (2016, fig. 5). Art © The Right Rehab, LLC.

Mental Disorders

Since addiction is a disease of the brain, it frequently occurs with other mental disorders. The question is, then, which disorder is driving the other? Does the mental disorder(s) drive the substance use to minimize its effects, or does the substance use drive or induce the mental disorder? Either way, today's research indicates that both illnesses should be treated in an integrated fashion.

But what do the doctors mean by the term *mental disorder?* In layman's terms, mental illness or disorders are generally characterized by changes in mood or thought that range from mild to severe. Anxiety disorders are the most common type followed by depressive ones. The other common mental disorders include bipolar, schizophrenia, and dementia.

Generic mental illness is broken down into one broad category—any mental illness (AMI)—and a smaller one—serious mental illness (SMI). These categories are *not* mutually exclusive—AMI includes all mental disorders, while SMI is a more severe subset of AMI.

An adult having any mental, behavioral, or emotional disorder in the past year that ranges from none to mild impairment for two weeks or less all the way up to full-blown schizophrenia has an AMI. Adults with AMI are defined as having SMI if they have any mental, behavioral, or emotional disorder that substantially interferes with or limits one or more major life activities. Symptoms of SMI include the inability to work, function in school, interact with family, and fulfill other major life activities.[11]

Substance misuse attracts most of the attention in our world today—any illness that snuffs out more than seventy thousand lives within a year should. However, even with 51.5 million people suffering from mental illness—that's 20 percent of us eighteen years of age or older—ranging from mild to severe in our country today, the attention mental illness actually receives unjustly takes a back seat to drug addiction. This is shocking, especially when you consider that there are 9.5 million adults who have both a mental illness and SUD. And leaving mental illness untreated is shameful.

For those treatment facilities that treat co-occurring disorders, the most common mental disorders treated simultaneously include:

- Depression
- Anxiety/panic attacks
- Schizophrenia
- PTSD—experiential, emotional, physical, or sexual trauma
- Dissociative identity disorder (formerly known as multiple personality disorder)
- Borderline personality disorder
- Bipolar disorder
- Obsessive/compulsive behavior
- Impulse control
- Anger issues
- ADHD (attention-deficit hyperactivity disorder)
- Bulimia

It's not enough for someone to be diagnosed with a dual diagnosis or co-occurring disorder. "Okay, we'll just treat them simultaneously." No! In order to get the right treatment, it is key to know which is the primary and secondary of the two. That diagnosis can only be determined by a qualified, certified, and experienced health care professional licensed in that discipline. A patient whose illness is primary mental illness and secondary substance abuse has to get treatment at a facility whose licensure is exactly that.

This is also when knowing who and where the right facilities are is paramount. You don't send that individual to a facility that, as an afterthought, says, "Oh, yeah. We can treat that, too."

Process Addiction

Although drug and alcohol addiction suck up most of the oxygen, there are other addictions that are no less serious and are treated as diseases. Process addiction is an addictive behavior that does not necessarily involve substance misuse but is obsessive conduct that compels the individual to engage compulsively and repeatedly in behavior detrimental to the individual. Obsessive behaviors include the following:

- Gambling
- Sex and intimacy
- Love
- Pornography
- Work
- Compulsive buying/shopping
- Internet
- Eating disorder
- Self-harming—burning, cutting, hair pulling
- Codependency
- Gaming

Evidence-Based Treatment

"Treatment centers can only prepare patients to follow through with their ongoing recovery but can't do it for them."

—Debra Jay[12]

Evidence-based therapies are called "evidence based" because of the voluminous evidence of research and studies proving that these therapies build skills to resist substance use, as well as increase life skills to handle stressful circumstances and triggers to use. In other words, they work.

Individual therapy helps people develop coping strategies and tools to maintain abstinence. In therapy, people learn how to

- identify the problem and be motivated to change;
- provide incentives for abstinence;
- repair damaged relationships with family and friends;
- develop personal accountability and responsibility;

- build new friendships with people in recovery;
- replace substance-using activities with constructive and rewarding ones;
- improve problem-solving skills; and
- create a recovery lifestyle.

Group therapy provides social reinforcement through peer discussion and support of one another in the common struggle to maintain sobriety. The individual's own experiences, feelings, and problems are validated by those who are experiencing the same issues. This helps the person in recovery learn additional coping skills because he is not the only one to experience those feelings—the victim is not alone.

Cognitive behavioral therapy (CBT) is the most researched and evaluated of all the therapies used for SUD and mental disorder treatment since it focuses on identifying, understanding, and changing thinking and behavior patterns. Among other benefits, CBT helps people do the following:

- Quickly identify and develop coping strategies with specific situations or conditions in one's life.
- Manage and conquer negative feelings and fears.
- Improve in a relatively short time.
- Work in a collaborative, goal-oriented, and practical approach to problem solving.
- Be effective in individual or group sessions.

Additionally, CBT is effective when combined with medications.

Dialectical behavioral therapy (DBT), per its developers, Marsha M. Linehan, PhD, and Linda A. Dimeff, PhD, is "treatment for individuals with multiple and severe psychological disorders, including those who are chronically suicidal"[13] and "focuses on problem solving and acceptance-based strategies."[14] "It aims to help residents in a very specific, organized fashion and focuses on changing harmful behaviors. By focusing on facts rather than emotions or value judgments such as good/bad or fair/unfair, DBT residents enhance their abilities to respond positively and productively, without descending into self-blame or other destructive thoughts and behaviors."[15]

Matrix Model therapists are trained to develop a positive, non-confrontational relationship with the patient to reinforce positive behavior change. Critical is promoting the patient's self-esteem, dignity, and self-worth. It includes elements of relapse prevention, family and group therapies, drug education, and self-help participation.

Family behavioral therapy (FBT) helps the family understand the disease and its causes, effects, and treatment. It is especially critical in treatment for adolescents as a therapeutic approach addressing family issues including substance use, mental disorders, and family conflict.

Behavioral couples therapy (BCT) is probably the most studied and applied family therapy. BCT promotes a "daily sobriety contract" between the patient and his or her spouse in which the patient commits to abstinence and the spouse promises support for those efforts. BCT also helps with communication and promotes non-substance-related activities that couples can share. Its effectiveness has been proven by reduced social costs related to substance abuse and intimate partner violence.

Eye movement desensitization and reprocessing (EMDR) is extensively used for victims of trauma. The patient follows the back-and-forth movement of the therapist's fingers in front of the patient's face, which helps the patient process and try to make sense out of upsetting memories, thoughts, and feelings related to trauma and start to heal from their harmful effects.

Brainspotting is similar to EMDR. With the aid of a pointer, the therapist guides the patient's eyes to a particular spot that the patient associates with a traumatic event and activates the mind and body to start the healing process. It is a remarkably useful tool in treating severe PTSD.

Psychodrama is a method of psychotherapy in which patients act out their personal problems by spontaneously enacting specific roles in dramatic performances before fellow patients. Mostly used in group therapy, it enables the patient to better understand past and present experiences—and how past experiences influence their lives. Its clinical potency makes it a powerful potential for growth, but there is also equal potential for damage if poorly conducted.

(No kidding about it being a powerful tool. The one experience I had with psychodrama was an emotionally packed, real-life drama not only for the subject of the session but also for all members of the group. Have tissues handy. Impressive. Powerful. Emotional. Revealing.)

Medication-assisted therapy (MAT) combines behavioral therapies and FDA-approved medications, including methadone, buprenorphine, naltrexone, and vivitrol, to produce stable levels and eliminate uncontrollable cravings. Despite several treatment programs that strictly adhere to total abstinence and reject the use of any opioid-like medication, well-supported scientific evidence shows that when combined with evidence-based therapy, MAT reduces rates of relapse and deaths due to overdose.

Exposure therapy helps people face, control, and cope with their fear and feelings by gradually exposing them to the trauma they experienced—but in a safe manner by using imaging, writing, or even visiting the place where the event happened.

Equine therapy is also called equine-assisted therapy since it involves humans interacting with horses. Like humans, horses are social animals and have distinct behaviors and personalities. Benefits include helping the patient heal from trauma, improve communication skills, and establish healthy boundaries. By gaining the trust of the animal and building confidence working with it, the patient carries over those skills when interacting and establishing healthy relationships with people.

Relapse prevention helps the patient develop a prevention plan that includes learning the warning signs of relapse and the different skills to stay sober. It helps the recovering individual identify relapse triggers; cope with cravings; develop plans for handling stressful situations; and learn what to do if and when a relapse occurs.

Art therapy encourages an individual to creatively confront her traumatic issues through a nonverbal, visual manner—drawing, painting, or sculpture, for example—as opposed to just using language to communicate. Art therapy is especially useful with adolescents since a visual medium allows them to create visual metaphors for their feelings, fears, and stress.

Additional Treatment Techniques (Modalities)

Hypnotherapy is aimed at behavior modification by suggestion. It produces an altered state of consciousness and delves into the patient's unconscious mind. This therapy is to be led only by a trained, certified hypnotherapist.

Twelve-step programming includes on- and off-campus self-help, mutual-aid support groups that extend the effects of formal treatment. Most prominent is the Alcoholics Anonymous twelve-step model used in group therapy meetings that draws on the social support offered by peer discussion with the goal of sustaining a substance-free, lifelong recovery lifestyle.

Psycho-ed (or psychoeducational groups) educates patients about substance use and its consequences with the purpose of motivating their commitment to abstinence.

Additional services include the following:

- Drug or alcohol urine testing
- Screening for human immunodeficiency virus (HIV); tuberculosis (TB); hepatitis B and C; and sexually transmitted infections (STIs)
- Smoking cessation assistance

Fitness: If I have to explain why exercise helps the mind and body, you need a shrink.

Music therapy: Whether listening, writing, or playing it, music promotes healing in the brain damaged by drugs. It helps patients manage stress, cope with cravings, express their inner thoughts, and connect with others.

Holistic treatments include the following:

- Yoga unifies the mind and body and creates inner peace.
- Meditation clears the mind and develops a state of self-awareness.
- Acupuncture is proven to reduce cravings and increase retention rates.
- Massage increases endorphins and decreases stress.

Adventure/experiential therapy: From wilderness survival to a climbing wall, the goal of this nature-based therapy is to present the individual with a challenge outside of her normal comfort zone and teaches skills to overcome it. Individuals learn survival and coping skills; build self-reliance, self-esteem, and confidence; and develop interpersonal skills while at the same time improving physical and mental well-being. Depending on the rehab's location and the season, activities include the following:

- Outdoor survival
- Ropes course
- Climbing wall
- Backpacking
- Canoeing
- Rock climbing
- Zip-lining
- Hiking
- Camping
- Whitewater rafting
- Organized sports
- Fitness training
- Skiing and snowboarding
- Mountain biking

Nutritional counseling: Since substance abuse often leads to poor nutrition, disrupts metabolic regulation and nutrient processing, and introduces toxins into the body, a return to healthy nutrient consumption becomes a priority in aiding recovery.

Life skills classes: Sober life skills are behaviors and social skills a person in recovery will have to relearn. Before treatment, most of the victim's activities and relationships centered on obtaining and using drugs or alcohol. Individuals striving for recovery need to learn a whole new way to live and make new friends. Among other skills, these classes teach the following:

- Employment, social, and communication skills
- Anger, stress, money, and time management
- Healthy leisure activities to replace previous substance use
- Goal setting
- Budgeting
- Shopping economically

These classes also inform learners about available social services.

Education counseling: For those without a high school diploma, achieving a GED is mandatory at most treatment facilities. For those who wish to resume college or attend one for the first time, top facilities offer mentoring on which institution is a good fit and assist with applications and organizing transcripts.

Job search counseling helps the individuals figure out which field or career is a good fit. Facilitators teach how to write a resume, offer interview coaching, and help individuals form a plan so that employment and a sober lifestyle coexist.

Housing assistance helps individuals in securing sober living and a recovery lifestyle so they can live in an environment with others who promote and support their sobriety.

Childcare: Being aware of and accessing different resources available allows parents to attend job interviews and secure eventual employment.

Discharge planning: Before leaving the structured environment of the rehab, discharge planning arranges several services including the following:

- MAT-certified providers
- Psychologists and counselors for additional therapy
- Twelve-step meeting locations and schedules
- Federal, state, or local social services
- Sober living houses
- Childcare services
- Career and employment counseling

THE RIGHT REHAB

"I have other obligations in my life now—the show, my family, my life . . . though I know that without my sobriety I wouldn't have any of those things."

—Rob Lowe[1]

Which Is the Right One?

When I started working with families, I met with one family in my conference room—nine of them came for the meeting. I well remember one of the adult male members asking, "All I have to do is Google 'rehabs,' and I see hundreds of them out there. Why are we hiring you?"

"Actually, there's more than sixteen thousand of them out there," I replied. "Can you tell me which is the right one for your nephew?"

Awkward pause, and then: "Good point."

That is precisely why I do what I do and wrote this book.

Out of the 19,795 that call themselves treatment centers or "rehabs" in 2019, the Substance Abuse and Mental Health Services Administration (SAMHSA) surveyed 15,961 of them.[2] All you have to do is pick the right one for you or your loved one. Easy, right? The point is that if you've never done this before and know nothing about rehab, how do you do that?

One answer is to talk with someone who is in recovery. How did that person get sober? Did he go to rehab or just meetings? Could the person recommend a rehab or a meeting? A person in recovery could also recommend someone you could call or someone else who has been to rehab. You can call your doctor, lawyer, church, or synagogue. Try a hospital ER; they usually have a list of local treatment facilities—mostly outpatient—likely faded since it's been copied a thousand times and probably needs updating.

An always reliable source of ethical treatment programs and facilities is the National Association of Addiction Treatment Professionals (NAATP). Known as the voice of the highest quality treatment professionals in the United States as well as being their voice on Capitol Hill, the NAATP holds its members to high ethical standards. The organization may be reached at 1-888-574-1008, or visit the website at https://www.naatp.org/.

One Size Does *Not* Fit All

The key is finding the right rehab for each individual. It's one thing to have the name of a facility, but is it the right one for that particular individual? To determine that, you've got to get into the details of the individual's diagnosis and several factors particular to the patient, and then match the patient with the facility that best fits the person's profile.

In the simplest of definitions, formal treatment at a reputable facility typically incorporates a combination of detox, behavioral therapies, and medications; the facility then structures an aftercare plan or—recovery support services (RSS)—when the individual is transitioning into "the real world." However, no one treatment facility or one single treatment is "the right one" for every individual and disorder.

The key is finding the right rehab for each individual. It's one thing to have the name of a facility, but is it the right one for that particular person? For that, you've got to get into the details of the individual's diagnosis and several factors particular to the patient, then match the patient with the facility that best fits her profile.

Variables include the following:

- DOC: Drug(s) of choice
- Co-occurring disorder (if one is diagnosed)
- Drug-related and other medical issues
- Goals and milestones (and steps to achieve them)
- Age, race and ethnicity
- Sexual orientation
- Gender identity
- Economic and social status
- Vocation
- Language
- Health literacy
- Legal problems
- Financial and/or insurance resources

For my clients, I formulate a one-year treatment plan. However, once a facility is chosen, that facility and therapists working with my client take precedence over deciding the best aftercare plan for the client. After all, they are the trained and certified treatment professionals who have the long-term therapeutic experience with my client that I will never have. They are the best qualified to determine the continuum of care that is personalized and attends to the multiple needs particular to that patient. My role then is to assist and implement that plan and work with my client for at least the balance of a year or more.

Here's one reason I love working with facilities that have integrity—the ones that value the patient's welfare as the primary mission. If they don't feel they are the best place for that particular individual, they routinely refer me to other rehabs—and will even call them for me. The "good guys" in this business all know and respect each other. They don't see other rehabs as competition—they see that what's good for one facility is good for all of them. The rehabs that promise anything just to get your business are the outliers, and the real pros know who they are.

When a client hires me, I work with the mantra "no surprises." My job is to determine the facility with the best treatment options available based on the individual's variables I mentioned earlier. Once I have determined the facilities that are the best fit, I then make all the arrangements—including financial—for admission at each one so all that's left is for the client to say yes or no. That includes making the best deal for my client, as well as detailing exactly what fees the client is expected to pay.

The client has enough to think about without having to figure out the best facility and then make all the arrangements. I make sure there are no surprises later. There are only two items I cannot do myself: the over-the-phone assessment between the patient and a facility clinician and the confirmation of resources between the financial guarantor and the facility.

Some of the stories clients tell me about their experiences with unethical facilities before they came to me are true nightmares. Michael, who stayed in a sober living house for seven months in southern California, had one outpatient group session per week, and yet the facility managed to wrangle $90,000 out of his insurance company for bogus and overpriced drug testing, as well as treatment sessions that never occurred.

Then there's David, whose wife went to alcohol treatment at a facility in southern Florida. Although he was promised that his upfront $6,700 payment, plus insurance benefits, would cover the entire thirty days of treatment, it didn't stop the facility from hitting him with a $15,000 bill upon her return home. The rehab claimed that her insurance company's payments didn't come close to covering their billing rate and other costs, so they billed him for the balance. Welcome to "balance billing," where rehabs set their own pricing, and when the insurance company doesn't meet that arbitrary price, they pass along to you the "balance of what they are owed."

Oh, and despite their promise to David that they were in-network with his insurance company, they weren't.

The point is, like so many other business sectors, there are charlatans who prey upon the vulnerabilities of families hit by addiction to make a quick buck. That's why people call someone like me to steer them clear of the "bad guys" and go to the right rehab for their particular situation.

Anytime you are told by a treatment facility—either in a cold call from a call center or on the other end of a toll-free number flashing on your late-night TV screen—that they are the right facility since they treat everything, hang up and block their number. No such rehab exists on this planet. Period.

Avoid the Following

In order to make the optimum choice for you or your loved one, you have to know the options that best fit the needs of the individual, plus the resources available to pay for them.

Let's start with scenarios and facilities that you should avoid:

- TV commercials that direct you to call a toll-free number. Your call actually goes to a call center packed with "treatment specialists" desperately trying to close sales with people just like you. They are not treatment specialists; they're sales representatives reading from a script peddling as many open beds as possible. And if you call back and wish to speak with the same representative again, good luck—the chances of you speaking with the same representative again are nil.
- Body brokering. A "treatment specialist" pumps you for insurance, financial, and extremely personal information that is going into their database. With that "assessment," they then auction your treatment to one or more rehabs in return for a referral fee, but they don't tell you that. Their service is tempting at first since it is free of charge to you. However,

you don't know whether the company is recommending a specific rehab because it is the best treatment for you or your loved one or because is it the one paying the highest commission. This "body-brokering" approach is dishonest and unethical, and in some states, it's illegal.

- Aggressive sales representatives who offer to pay for your flight—one way, of course.
- Facilities that say they accept your insurance. Confirm it. What they often don't tell you is whether they are an in-network or out-of-network facility. "Out-of-network" means that the deductible, out-of-pocket maximum and treatment reimbursement rates are higher in the rehab's favor—frequently double what they would be at an in-network facility. Plus, instead of asking for those fees upfront—which is normal practice at ethical facilities—frequently they squeeze you for them later when you are already in treatment, causing you to panic that you'll be kicked out unless you come up with the cash. If you don't have it, they either kick you out or bill you, making you legally liable for the fees. And it doesn't end there. Some of these outfits actually sic a collection agency on you and ruin your credit along with it. I can tell you horror stories of victims with less than thirty days of treatment who have been escorted off the rehab property when their insurance company stops authorizing payments and they didn't have the ability to pay cash for the rest of their treatment. Ethical rehabs don't do that.
- Rehabs that won't confirm the costs quoted to you over the phone via e-mail or fax.
- Facilities that don't disclose additional fees they charge separately for sessions with a psychiatrist or a physician, medications, and local transportation.
- A facility unknown to long-time treatment professionals.
- Rehabs that are not certified by CARF International (the Commission on Accreditation of Rehabilitation Facilities)

or the Joint Commission. Both are nonprofit accreditors of health care service providers. Between the two, they certify more than twenty-eight thousand providers domestically and worldwide.

- Rehabs that are not members of the National Association of Addiction Treatment Providers (NAATP), the ultimate umpire of ethical treatment practices. If a facility violates NAATP's code of ethics, it's called out and possibly expelled.
- Be wary of those owned by equity or hedge funds. Most of them are in it for the return on their investment, not optimum treatment for the individual.
- A rehab that recently changed its name and corporate identity. That could be a sign that the facility has been sued, went bankrupt, or abruptly changed ownership for a suspicious reason.

Know the Following

Obviously, you want to pick the treatment facility that is the best fit for you or your loved one's needs. You will want to know the following before making that judgment. Do you want to drive a 1-800 sales representative crazy? Ask the rep the following questions:

The Facility Itself

→ Is there a renowned staff member, consultant, or treatment program that enhances the facility's reputation? What is the facility known to excel at (and respected for)? Does the facility have expertise in dealing with a specific area (e.g., trauma, reactive attachment disorder [RAD], veterans, equine therapy, wilderness track, sex addiction, eating disorders, etc.)? Is there a professional track for executives (e.g., lawyers, doctors, first responders)? If so, are any of them stand-alone programs?

➔ Are you deciding on a particular facility because it is the best fit with the individual's diagnosis or because it is the most convenient to reach for the family?

➔ Is the facility state certified? Has it ever been sanctioned or had its license suspended? Is its license still active?

➔ Are you receiving a referral fee?

➔ What is the facility's licensure?
  ◆ Substance abuse (SA)?
  ◆ Mental health (MH)?
  ◆ Primary SA + secondary MH?
  ◆ Primary MH + secondary SA?
  ◆ Primary MH + primary SA?

➔ Who owns the facility?
  ◆ How many years has it been operating?
  ◆ Who started it and why?
  ◆ Is it privately owned?
  ◆ Is the owner a person, family, or a group of individuals who are in recovery themselves?
  ◆ Did the owner get sober there and decide to buy it?
  ◆ Is the facility owned by a foundation?
  ◆ Is it a nonprofit?
  ◆ Is the facility owned by an equity or hedge fund?
  ◆ Is it owned by a health care company?
  ◆ Is it publicly owned?
  ◆ Has the facility changed hands, and if so, how many times?
  ◆ Do the executives who run it have experience running a treatment facility?

➔ Is there an active alumni group?

➔ Does the facility offer references?

➔ Does the facility offer any studies or metrics on the sobriety rates of their clients one year after discharge?

➔ Which demographics does the facility serve?
  ◆ Adolescents (twelve to seventeen)?

- ◆ Young adults (eighteen to twenty-five)?
- ◆ Adults (twenty-six and older)?
- ◆ Seniors?
- ◆ Veterans?
- ◆ State-sponsored clientele?
- ◆ Court-ordered clientele?
- ◆ Professional track clientele (doctors, lawyers, pilots, first responders, etc.)?
- ◆ Faith-based clientele?
- ◆ Single-sex clientele?
- ◆ Coed clientele?
- ◆ Coed clientele with gender-specific therapy?
- ◆ LGBT/transgender clientele?
→ What is the facility's population?
- ◆ What is the facility's capacity?
- ◆ What is the age range of the current population?
- ◆ What is the current number of males? Females?
- ◆ What is the current gender ratio?
- ◆ What regions of the country are represented?
- ◆ Are there any international patients?
→ What is the ALS (average length of stay)?
- ◆ Thirty days?
- ◆ Forty-five days?
- ◆ Sixty days?
- ◆ Ninety days?
- ◆ Six, nine, or twelve months?
→ Does the facility create a one-year treatment plan for the individual that includes formal treatment followed by long-term aftercare?
→ What is the distance to the nearest hospital emergency room?
→ What security protocols are in place?
- ◆ How secure are the patients from public access?
- ◆ How stringently is the rehab enforcing HIPAA guidelines regarding callers and visitors?

◆ Does the facility assign an access "code" that identifies friends and family with permission to speak with the patient and get status updates?

→ What are the facility grounds like?

  ◆ What is the size of the campus?
  ◆ What is the setting?
    • Urban?
    • Rural?
    • Suburban?
    • Residential neighborhood?

Paying for Treatment

→ How is treatment paid?

  ◆ Insurance
    • Is the facility in-network with any insurance companies?
    • If yes, with which insurance companies is it in-network?
    • If it's an out-of-network facility, will the facility still file for out-of-network benefits during or after treatment?
    • Will the facility confirm where insurance payments are to be sent—to the facility or to you, the insured?
    • Do they accept
      ○ Medicare?
      ○ Medicaid?
      ○ TriCare?
      ○ CHAMP/VA or CHAMP/US?
    • Does the facility need the remainder of your deductible and out-of-pocket maximum paid upfront?
    • Will the facility accept a payment schedule for that upfront amount?
    • Does the facility require a deposit for future room and board fees when the patient steps down to partial

hospitalization programming (PHP) from residential care and bifurcate the billing?
- Will the facility confirm the deal in writing?

◆ Private pay
- What does the facility charge per day? Per month? For three months?
- Does the facility offer a discount for total paid upfront?
- Does the facility discount subsequent monthly fees after the first one or two months?
- Will the facility accept a payment plan?
- Will the facility refer the patient to loan companies, if necessary?
- Does the facility offer scholarships?
- Will the facility confirm the deal in writing?

→ Are there additional fees?
◆ Are medications included in the overall fee, or are these charged separately?
◆ Does the patient need to post a retainer or deposit for medications?
◆ Does the facility have an on-site pharmacy?
◆ If there's no on-site pharmacy, does the patient need to set up an account at an off-site pharmacy?
◆ Is a debit card the preferred manner to send the patient spending money for off-site meals, shopping, and such?
◆ Does the facility charge separate fees for sessions with a psychiatrist and physician?

Modalities

→ Are these evidence-based therapies available?
◆ CBT (cognitive behavioral therapy)
◆ DBT (dialectical behavioral therapy)
◆ Contingency management

- FBT (family behavioral therapy)
- BCT (behavioral couples therapy)
- EMDR (eye movement desensitization and reprocessing)
- Brainspotting
- Psychodrama
- Exposure therapy
- Relapse prevention
- Art therapy
- Music therapy
- Equine therapy
- Twelve-step meetings (on- and off-campus)
- Hypnotherapy
- Psycho-ed
- Adventure/experiential therapy

→ What is the facility's position on medication-assisted therapy (MAT)?

→ Does the facility offer holistic treatment?
- Yoga
- Meditation
- Acupuncture
- Massage
- Nutrition counseling

→ What other programs does the facility offer?
- Fitness
- Life skills classes
- GED or other continuing education classes
- Employment counseling sessions

Caregivers

→ What is the facility's staff like?
- What's the combined average years of practice?
  - Are there a psychiatrist and a physician on staff?
  - How many therapists and counselors are on the staff?

- Are the treatment personnel employees or contractors?
- How many individual sessions (with a psychiatrist, physician, or counselor) per week are allocated to each patient?
- Are there additional sessions available with or without additional charge?
- What's the counselor-to-patient ratio?
- How many of the therapists have a master's degree?
- How many and what types of licenses do the therapists and counselors have?
- What's the composition of night duty staff?
- Is a nurse on the premises 24/7?

Facility Policies

→ What are the facility's policies regarding nutrition and housekeeping?
- ◆ Are the meals planned and prepared by a chef or a staff dietician?
- ◆ Do patients do their own shopping and prepare their own meals?
- ◆ Is there maid service for heavy cleaning of patient rooms?
- ◆ Are patients expected to do light housekeeping?
- ◆ Are they expected to make their beds daily?
- ◆ Are they expected to bring their own towels and bedding?
- ◆ Are they expected to do their own laundry, or is it sent out?
- ◆ Does the facility offer laundry supplies, or do patients shop for them?

→ What is the facility's policy on smoking?
- ◆ Is smoking allowed? Prohibited?
- ◆ Is smoking allowed in designated areas?
- ◆ Is smoking regulated by a schedule?

→ What is the facility's policy on visitation?
- ◆ Is it family only?

- ◆ Are friends allowed?
- ◆ Are visits allowed during the week or on weekends only?
- ◆ Are visits prohibited during the first weeks of the patient's stay?
- ◆ How much advance notice is necessary?
- → What is the facility's policy on phone and computer use?
  - ◆ Is there a probation period?
  - ◆ Are phone calls only permitted on a monitored landline?
  - ◆ Are there time restrictions on phone use?
  - ◆ Are there restrictions on cell phone use?
  - ◆ Are there restrictions regarding computers?
- → What is the facility's policy on contraband?
  - ◆ Ahead of admission, does the facility send a list of recommended clothing and items prohibited and allowed?
  - ◆ Do staff perform a thorough search of the person and belongings with every new admittance?
  - ◆ Do staff perform unannounced, random room searches? How often?
  - ◆ What happens if contraband is discovered?
  - ◆ How often does the facility administer drug tests?
  - ◆ What happens when there is a positive test result?

Treatment Stages

- → How does the facility handle detox?
  - ◆ Does the facility have its own detox unit?
  - ◆ Is the unit on or off campus?
  - ◆ Is detox done at an off-site contractor, a hospital, or a non-hospital facility?
  - ◆ Are the services billed through the rehab or directly from the detox unit?
  - ◆ Are detox days counted as part of residential treatment?
- → What does the facility's residential treatment program look like?

- ◆ What is the facility's average length of stay (ALS)?
- ◆ What is its daily schedule?
- ◆ What is the setting?
  - Is it a hospital-type setting?
    - ○ Dormitory?
    - ○ Cottage?
    - ○ Residential home?
    - ○ Single room?
    - ○ Are there two patients or more per room?
  - What treatment components are administered off-campus?
- ◆ What has been the average number of days authorized for residential care recently by the insurance company?
- ◆ When your insurance company ends authorizing residential days, does the insurance company step the patient down to partial hospitalization programming (PHP)?
- ◆ When step-down to PHP occurs, does the facility bifurcate the billing and keep the patient in the residential setting until day 30, or do they move the patient to sober living prior to day 30?
  - Does the facility bill the patient for room and board?
  - What is the daily rate?
  - Is an upfront deposit mandatory?
  - Does the facility absorb the room and board and not bill the patient separately for it?
- → What does the facility's partial hospitalization programming (PHP) look like?
  - ◆ What has been the average number of days/sessions authorized by the insurance company for a PHP recently?
    - Five days per week?
    - Six or eight hours per day?
  - ◆ Does the patient continue residing in the residential setting during the entire PHP or move to a sober living environment after day 30?

→ What does the facility's intensive outpatient programming (IOP) and outpatient programming (OP) look like?
- Does the facility have its own program?
- Is treatment on or off-site?
- Is treatment provided by a separate contractor?
- Is treatment offered by a sober living facility as part of its program?
- Does the program start at five sessions per week and step down to three?
- What is the length of each session?
- Are the sessions all gender specific or all coed?
- How many patients are there per session?
- What's the average number of sessions authorized by your insurance?
- Does the program offer morning and evening sessions?
- Does the patient move to a sober living house or apartment?
- Does the facility provide transportation to and from the IOP?
- When can the patient schedule employment, education, or community service when not in therapy?

→ What does the facility offer regarding sober living accommodations?
- What's the capacity of the sober living facility?
- Is the sober living facility owned by the treatment facility?
- Is the sober living facility a house, apartment, or dormitory?
- Is sober living provided by an independent contractor?
- If sober living is provided by an independent contractor, what is the length of the relationship with the facility?
- How are services billed?
- What's the monthly rate?
- What's the average number of weeks, months, or years residents stay?
- Does the sober living facility allow medication-assisted therapy?

- How far is the sober living facility from the IOP and OP treatment locations?
- Does the sober living facility provide transportation to and from treatment locations?
- How accessible is public transportation?
- What is the drug-testing policy?
- What happens if there is a positive test?
- Are there random room searches?
- What happens if contraband is discovered?
- Which chores are mandatory?
- What is the sober living facility's policy on resident employment, education, or community service?
- How many twelve-step meetings are mandatory per week?
- Does the sober living facility host twelve-step meetings?
- If not, is there transportation to and from twelve-step meetings?
- Is there a resident car policy?
- What is the curfew policy?
- What is the policy on overnight stays outside of the sober living facility?

Continuum of Care/Aftercare/Maintenance

→ What does the facility's continuum of care look like?
- Does the facility put in place a separate aftercare plan for millennials and older adults?
- Does the facility encourage the patient to start a new, sober life locally or somewhere other than the patient's hometown (especially for millennials)?
- Is the sober living environment available for the balance of the year or longer if required?
- Are there twelve-step meetings and other mutual-aid support groups and activities?
- Is there an alumni group?

- ◆ Are there fitness options?
- ◆ Are there options for outpatient treatment and individual therapy?
- ◆ Will the facility set the patient up with an approved physician if MAT is part of the plan?
- ◆ Are career and job counseling available?
- ◆ Is education counseling available?
- ◆ Are childcare services available?
- ◆ Is there financial, budget, and banking counseling available?
- ◆ Are legal services available?
- ◆ If the patient is staying in new location, does the facility encourage the patient not to return home for at least one year and to make the visit as short as possible?

Now that we have reviewed what treatment is and components of the right rehab, we move on to getting the patient to that rehab.

INTERVENTION

"Rock bottom became the solid foundation on which I rebuilt my life."

—J. K. Rowling[1]

"Enablement is what allows the victim to continue using. Intervention is what we do to stop enablement."

—Walter Wolf

People stop using substances for various reasons. If it is the threat of incarceration, well, that's easy—go to rehab or go to the slammer. Sending the individual to rehab immediately (if possible, before charges are filed) doesn't guarantee non-incarceration; however, sending an offender to rehab as part of a one-year treatment plan right after the arrest goes a long way in postponing the arraignment and softening the eventual outcome for the defendant.

In order to be successful, there must be coordination among the defense attorney, the district attorney (DA), the judge, and, of course, the defendant. In the countless times I have been a part of this process for nonviolent offenders, judges and DAs have always been agreeable to the defendant getting treatment as opposed to imposing incarceration.

Other motivations to stop using include loss or impending loss of a job; a spouse and/or family's threat to leave; loss of home, friends, or money; and even, sadly, death—whatever it takes for someone to "hit bottom." I have had clients go to treatment and remain sober to this day for those reasons and, unfortunately, a few who didn't.

Intervention is normally the last thing the individual is expecting, and he is usually not too accommodating. Probably the easiest is intervening between an adult child living at home and the family members enabling the adult child to continue the substance abuse. As long as the enablement continues, nothing is going to change. Frequently, the hardest part of the intervention is getting the family members to follow through on their commitment to cut their loved one off and not enable further in a moment of weakness or because of guilt.

There are two dominant forms of intervention: first, changing the family's interaction with the individual to gradually achieve the loved one's surrender to treatment, and second, a family's direct confrontation with the family member—"Go to treatment now or else . . ."

Behind door number 1 is the highly regarded CRAFT (Community Reinforcement Approach to Family Training) system. Chiefly developed by Robert Meyers, PhD, at the University of New Mexico, CRAFT teaches family members how to—in a non-confrontational way—"break your unintentional participation in patterns related to their loved-one's use. For example, a mother who often calls her son's employer to say that he is too sick to come into work, when he is really too hungover to come into work, will stop making those calls. Instead, she will calmly express that she is no longer willing to call in sick for her son."[2]

The positive factor of CRAFT is that the family's progressive, consistent, non-enabling behavior frequently produces the "Hey, I gotta stop this shit or I'm gonna die" moment when the individual finally surrenders and goes to treatment because she chooses to go. On the negative side, it often takes time for CRAFT to be effective, and frequently the family's patience breaks down before success can be achieved. The unspoken fear, of course, is that the addiction will lead to a criminal justice nightmare or, even worse, kill the individual before that goal can be achieved. Is the family willing to take that chance?

If the family is simply too exhausted to invest more time trying to get their loved one to treatment, and they fear an impending train wreck, that's when it's time for door number 2. I learned this form of intervention from a renowned treatment professional, Mike Early, who gained unparalleled experience and knowledge through literally fifty years of sobriety. Mike has worked with treatment facilities of the highest quality, ethics, and reputations, including Hazelden in Minnesota, Caron Foundation in Pennsylvania, and Northbound Treatment Center in Southern California. Just when he thinks it's time to retire, his skills and experience are inexorably needed. Mike reminds me of Michael Corleone in *The Godfather Part III*: "Just when I thought I was out, they pull me back in."

Mike's method of intervention is the same one that worked on him fifty years ago. It's remarkably simple—find the source of the individual's enablement and cut it off. Something or someone is enabling the victim to continue being addicted, and it has got to come to a screeching halt. Give the individual two choices: "Go immediately to rehab, or get in the car and we'll find you a new home under a bridge."

Does it work every time? No—but name one treatment that does. Tragically, there are those souls whose addiction is so embedded and so chronic that eventual death is their only "cure."

The first step in working with a family who wants a noncompliant family member to go to rehab is knowing the DOC (drug of choice). From where and whom does the individual get it? How does he pay for it? Does he use it at home or away? How long has this been going on? There are other issues to consider. Is there a diagnosis from a medical provider? Does he have a co-occurring mental disorder or history of trauma? Has he ever been to treatment? Has he been to an ER, physician, therapist, counselor, or substance treatment recently? Do any family members have consent to speak with a professional who has treated him? Are medical records available? Are there criminal justice issues? Does he have an attorney, and does that attorney have consent to speak with a family member? If there is no attorney, does he need one?

If legal issues are involved, and if there isn't one already, hiring an attorney is essential. Parents who hire an attorney for their adult child—or, for that matter, anyone else who hires an attorney for a family member—frequently make the mistake of believing that the attorney works for them (the payer of the fees). I've witnessed many upset parents and financial guarantors when they learn that the attorney works for the client—the subject—not the one who's paying the bill. As with medical issues, consent may be arranged, but that should be done upfront—not later when complicating issues could develop.

The next step is to determine the source of enablement. Who and what is making it possible for the victim to continue the addiction?

The Choice

> "Addiction is a family disease. One person may use, but the whole family suffers."
>
> —Shelly Lewis[3]

Here's a common situation that could easily be yours: an unemployed adult child is still living in the parents' home. Let's assume we have a son who has a roof over his head, food in the fridge, a car for transportation, a cell phone, and endless excuses to have access to cash—all while still getting high. Why should the individual change? All his needs are being met. If the child is dependent on the parents or other family members for this lifestyle, that's an easy one to stop. At the end of the day, intervention is all about cutting off the enablement.

And although the parents beg him to stop using drugs and cry out that they can no longer endure seeing their son destroy himself, their desperate pleading doesn't make a difference. When they threaten to stop paying for certain items unless he "straightens up," he knows these are idle threats, and, for good measure, that's when he plays the guilt card: "I swear I'm trying to get a job, but if you stop paying for my phone, how am I going to find one? If you take the car away, how am I supposed to get to job interviews?"

It's the classic standoff. Addiction does everything it can to defend itself. If it means walking all over the ones who love you, so be it. The addiction doesn't care.

A client of mine who relapsed several times before regaining recovery for the past three years described to me addiction's relentless hold on him: "After two weeks of sobriety and having a great job . . . everything was fine and then a thought popped in my head—getting high right now sounds great. That's when I went to a Walgreens parking lot and overdosed. . . . The ambulance showed up, and the first person I saw looking down at me in that ER was my mother, who I put through hell. She was there with tears in her eyes just begging me to change, and all I could think about was how can I get out of there before I have to go and face the music in court, to get that one last high."

> "When an alcoholic hits bottom, the family usually does, too."
>
> —Debra Jay[4]

Any semblance of a family life has been destroyed long ago, thanks to addiction. Family holidays and celebrations become hopelessly strained or don't happen anymore. Siblings blame the parents for enabling their brother to continue his life of destruction and have given up any hope of his resurrection. The parents hold on to a hopeless fantasy that one day he will just wake up, decide to stop using, and get his life together.

There's a scene in *Chinatown* (1974) when Jack Nicholson's character, a frustrated "J. J. Gittes," is trying to get Faye Dunaway's "Evelyn Mulwray" to reveal a dark family secret. With each of Gittes's slaps across Mulwray's face (a felony in today's world and never advised no matter how frustrating the situation), she blurts out, "She's my daughter." Slap! "She's my sister." Slap! "She's my daughter." Slap! "She's my sister." Slap! Now you know what it's like dealing with someone addicted who repeatedly says she wants to go to treatment but then says, "Nah, I can do this on my own" (minus the slapping, of course).

While most of us would call it "fucking crazy," the professionals who work in this field call it the "Transtheoretical Model of Change." Yes, they have noticed that behavior, too, but have a much more civilized and intelligent way of describing it than, say, me. Figure 4.1 depicts the process in visual terms.

Notice that the arrows in this figure signify that this process can go around and around, and the individual can go back and forth between stages unless and until the victim decides it's time to get off this merry-go-round of destruction and get sober.

As the figure shows, in the *precontemplation* stage the victim is unaware of the problem or at least acts as if there is not one. Either way, the victim is unwilling to do something about it or is too discouraged to do so.

In the *contemplation* stage, the victim expresses a desire to change but has no definite plans to do so. The two desires exist side by side—the desire to change and the desire to continue the current behavior (hence the *Chinatown* reference).

In the *preparation* stage, the individual is aware that her substance use is a problem and has made a conscious decision to change. If and when this occurs, action has to be taken immediately so that the individual doesn't change her mind.

In the *action* stage, the victim is actively in treatment.

During the *maintenance* stage, the victim is in remission and following an aftercare plan that includes sober living and mutual-aid

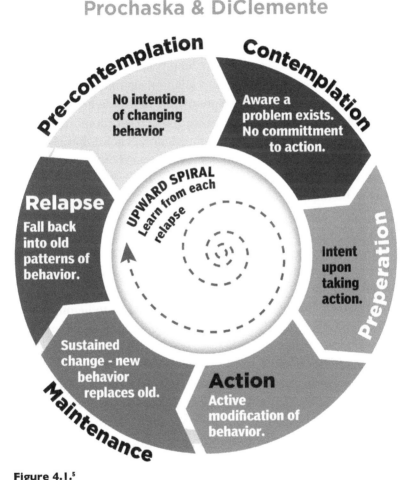

Transtheoretical Model of Change

Prochaska & DiClemente

Pre-contemplation
No intention of changing behavior

Contemplation
Aware a problem exists. No committment to action.

Preperation
Intent upon taking action.

Action
Active modification of behavior.

Maintenance
Sustained change - new behavior replaces old.

Relapse
Fall back into old patterns of behavior.

UPWARD SPIRAL
Learn from each relapse

Figure 4.1.[5]
Art © The Right Rehab, LLC.

support groups. The goal is to live a recovery lifestyle, which normally takes years, depending on any relapses along the way.

If there is *relapse*, this indicates a need to change some components of treatment, not that treatment has been a failure. Relapse is frequently part of the journey to recovery.

So far, I have described what millions of families are experiencing throughout our nation, but there is a light at the end of this tortuous tunnel. It begins with the family accepting that their enablement is feeding the disease and killing their child or loved one. What they must do is counterintuitive to most parents' instincts, but the plan will only work if they are 100 percent committed to it.

That's the hard part, offering the victim a choice, but sticking with the commitment to go through with either choice: "Accept our gift of treatment or pack your shit and go!" There is no negotiating. It has to be this plan, or all enablement stops *now*. Only when the individual is convinced that you mean what you say will it have the desired effect. "We've had enough of watching you kill yourself and our role in helping you do it. If you accept our offer of treatment and recovery, we pledge to do everything in our power to help and support you, but we cannot support any other choice."

At twenty-four, Karin was chronically addicted to heroin. Now a friend and colleague, she recounted for me when her mother, embittered by the failure of everything they had tried to make Karin stop, took her on a tour of local bridges so she could decide which one she would pick as her next home—which was to be the next step unless she decided to go to treatment. Today, she is a mother of a six-year-old boy and an executive for one of the most successful treatment providers in the country. Karin chose wisely.

When the Intervention Works

If the individual realizes that he cannot go on any longer and surrenders, the intervention is successful. But hold on, we're not done yet—the treatment plan must go into effect that nanosecond. Sometimes the intervention is the smoothest piece of the operation compared to the logistics of getting the victim there.

Time is the enemy. You want to get the individual out the door and into rehab as soon as possible, not later when she has time to change her mind or wants to see the other choices or, worse, research more options. That's why arrangements with the rehab have to occur prior to the intervention—the less the victim has to say about where she is going, the better. Don't invite her opinion, just get her there.

If the intervention is happening out of the family home, a family member should have surreptitiously packed a bag with rehab-approved clothes and items that are all ready to go. Just pack enough for the first couple of days. Yes, there will be items the individual will still want and need, but they can be shipped later, or he can purchase them on location. He can also phone in his goodbyes to friends while on the road or once he's there, depending on the facility's phone policy.

If travel by plane is necessary and the next day is the soonest flights are available, keep the victim at home, but have someone with the individual at all times. Do not let him out of the house alone or out of your sight.

If the victim is in the early stages of withdrawal or will be by travel time, if necessary, take him to a nearby detox facility for medical detoxification, which could last up to ten days. It's not a great choice since it is preferable for the long-term rehab to treat the patient from the beginning. Most important, you want to avoid the "miracle cure." That's when the victim is "clean" on the other side of withdrawal. She suddenly believes that she is "cured" and no longer needs to go to treatment. Along with the predictable return to her previous ways, there is the increased danger of death by overdose due to the victim's reduced tolerance to what she was previously ingesting.

If a medical caregiver is already involved with the patient, avoid a detox facility altogether by having medications ready for easing the symptoms just long enough for the journey per the particular substance of choice.

The point is to get the individual out the door as soon as possible, and if that means a multi-hour drive, so be it. As a veteran of these on-the-road journeys, I'll suggest certain items you'll want to have already prepared since you want to stop only for gas and bathroom breaks: a cooler for liquids and perishable food; sandwiches and snacks; a thermos for hot liquids; Starbucks VIA instant coffee, so all you'll need is hot water for coffee when you stop for gas; paper towels; Clorox disinfectant wipes; "barf" bags; and an absorbent blanket on the passenger seat for—well, you know.

During these long drives, I've noticed something peculiar about my fellow travelers. By the end of the journey, they no longer hate me. Frequently they detest me because I, as the interventionist, am the one disrupting their lives. It's sometimes quite educational learning new expressions of venom and hostility. Somewhere along the journey, however, there's a metamorphosis. They start to open up and admit they need to put an end to this disease, and they actually look forward to rebooting their lives and having a chance to start over.

It's surprisingly easy. All it really takes on my part is asking some questions about them: "So, Jamie, what's the least satisfactory part of your life? What do you wish to change?" And wham! They don't want to stop talking, nor should you try to stop them. The key is being a good listener, and you'll witness someone having a huge rock lifted off their chest. You can literally feel the relief. They've spent so much of their lives being told what to do instead of being asked what they want—and they feel someone is actually listening to them.

The payoff is at the end of the journey. The person who only hours earlier hated me with all his vitriol gives me a hug when entering intake.

This brings me to the next point about the person accompanying the individual—the escort. Generally, it's not a good idea for that person to be a parent or sometimes even a family member in order to avoid what I call the "scorecard." It goes like this:

> Parent: "You know, if you weren't such a fuck-up, I wouldn't be spending all our money on you!"
>
> Patient: "You know, if you weren't such a fucked-up parent, I wouldn't be a fucking addict!"

Even a watered-down version of this conversation can be difficult for parent and patient. You get it. It's not the ideal way to start a new life.

The point is that recovery starts the moment the individual is out the door. The last thing needed is for the victim to start a new life in a state of anger, when acting out is possible—and likely. Most of the time, I'm the one accompanying the individual to treatment since it is crucial to have a neutral party or a professional sober escort personally hand over the individual to the rehab in order to avoid the deep-seated, family-oriented acrimony.

Another reason for a neutral party is the over-the-phone assessment between the rehab and the individual. Although the rehab has had relevant information or medical records (if available per the Health Insurance Portability and Accountability Act [HIPPA]) on the soon-to-be patient prior to the intervention, most facilities need an assessment over the phone with the patient to prepare for the arrival and start devising a detailed treatment plan. It is crucial that the individual be completely honest and truthful about her drug use—I mean everything. Confessing those details in the presence of a parent or family member often constrains her truthfulness. That's not a good thing, especially if the treatment is insurance dependent since the insurance company's authorization of the several levels of treatment necessary is dependent on the individual's actual drug use. That assessment in the presence of a neutral third party removes those constraints.

Millennials

Here are some typical behavioral traits of some, not all, millennials—male and female—who needed an intervention to get them to treatment. Despite a warm farewell, it's usually at the beginning of residential treatment when the venom of resentment again raises its ugly self.

They hate me. They hate the world. They hate the rehab. For the next four nights, there are the phone calls—you can set a clock by them.

"I hate this fucking place. How could you fucking leave me here?" "The counselors are idiots. The guys are mean to me." "Why am I here? I'm not the same as the others." "The food sucks." "I have nothing in common with the other girls here; they're fucking morons." "Group is stupid; it doesn't help me a bit. This is a waste of my parents' money." "The other girls are here for trauma, so why am I here?" "I want my dog here—that's nonnegotiable." "You have until this weekend to get me to another place!"

And the tears. Oh my God, the tears.

When I address these issues with my clients' counselors, they could set the phone down, make some coffee, come back, and not miss a thing. They've heard it all before. I also can predict how the counselors are going to respond, usually with "Just give it some time, Walter." But the best response was from Richard Dorn at Still Waters outside of Nashville, Tennessee, which runs favorite programs of mine for males and females: "That's okay, Walter. We're just going to show Ethan some more love."

After an average of four days of "get me outta here" phone calls, they magically stop. I'll never forget a month after that first tearful call from Ethan. I was on a rehab road trip inhaling a Five Guys burger in Tallahassee, Florida, when I got a call from Ethan: "Walt! I just want you to know that I love this place, and I love you. You saved my life." "I love the other guys here; they're my brothers." The "more love" worked. Ethan got it. He knew he needed to be there.

"It's the brotherhood and sisterhood, Walter," explained Heath Chitwood, executive director of Still Waters. "A community that is built on peer love teaches you to love yourself. Our residents learn that you are your brother's keeper."[6]

Then there are the rare ones who refuse to get it or are just not ready for sobriety.

Despite years of heroin abuse, twenty-four-year-old Carolyn was still a stunningly beautiful young woman. One morning as I was preparing to take a client to Cumberland Heights in Nashville, Carolyn's lawyer called and pleaded that I immediately pick her up and get her into a detox unit. I'd have to push back picking up my client a bit, but I could make it work.

Imagine now every cliché assigned to a den of heroin addicts. This was worse. It was dark and full of dopers and sickening odors, and I was painfully aware that my sudden presence was not welcome. My right hand tightened around the pepper spray hidden in my pocket. I discovered Carolyn in a bedroom with four males; they had just finished shooting dope. Upon announcing that her lawyer sent me, I got her to hurriedly gather some clothes and got out of there pronto.

Despite her lack of insurance and money, I took her to three detox units in the city that admit such cases, but not one of them would take her because she was not yet in withdrawal. The fact that she would be withdrawing within a few hours didn't make a difference. No shakes, no room at the inn. Shit! What was I going to do?

I was getting nervous. This was unexpected, and not part of the game plan. I certainly was not going to return her to where I found her. I had no choice: "Carolyn, ever been to Nashville?" Carolyn excitedly exclaimed, "Road trip? Let's go!" Man, I wished I had her attitude. I had no choice—Carolyn was coming along to Nashville with my other client and myself. I had no idea what to do with her. I needed time to figure something out.

During the drive, I was close to panic. She'd be going into withdrawal at any time, and I had no place to take her. I was desperate.

At a gas stop, I called my friend Walt Quinn at Cumberland Heights. "Walt! What the hell do I do? She has no money, no insurance. I need your help, please." Walt replied, "You know, your name came up at our board meeting last week. Let me see what I can do."

Upon arriving at Cumberland Heights, I got my client admitted into detox. So far, so good, but what about Carolyn? The director of admissions, Jana Mason, pulled me into an empty office. She told me they were giving Carolyn ninety days of treatment—a program that ordinarily cost at that time $39,000—at no charge.

Then I did something totally unexpected—something I had not done in decades. I burst into tears. Me, a grown man. Tears.

In this book, I write about working with only rehabs of the highest quality and integrity. I just described one—Cumberland Heights—thanks to Walt and Jana.

In my farewell to Carolyn, I explained that she was receiving a gift. I told her she might not know it now, but it would change her life and she would appreciate it later. "Please do good with it," I begged her.

Carolyn walked away from the program a week later. She wasn't ready to get sober.

"Pack Your Shit and Go" Therapy

If an addict is happy with you, you're probably enabling them. If an addict is mad at you, you're probably trying to save their life.[7]

Unfortunately, during an intervention, the victim's surrender and departure for treatment doesn't always occur, so you have to be prepared for the worst:

- The patient denies there's a problem: "I don't need rehab! I can stop anytime I want."
- The individual leaves the room in a fit of rage: "Fuck you! I can't believe you tricked me like this!"

- The individual offers cop-out excuses, proving that he has no intention of actually getting sober. He instead tries to placate his enablers: "Okay, but I'm not going to that rehab. I'll go to outpatient treatment and AA meetings every night, I promise . . . it'll save you money, too."

The addiction is defending itself, and you are being played. This is when it's imperative that the family stick to their original offer and hold their ground. No negotiating. It's their way or the highway. No other avenues will be considered. It has to be "go to treatment," or else it's "pack your shit and go!"

With more than two hundred successful interventions under his belt, Jeffrey Klein, executive director of Crownview Co-Occurring Institute in Oceanside, California, taught me that the "most important factor between success and failure in an intervention is the absolute unity—the 'united front'—among the other family members. Once I feel this front will 'hold the line,' we move to the next stage of the intervention—'containment'—which is like a plastic container with the individual inside, cut off from all forms of enabling outside of that container. If, for whatever reason, a family member or friend cannot hold the line, they put a crack in the container, and the loved one spills out, rendering this stage of the intervention a failure."

Klein continued: "When all other measures are exhausted and the loved one remains defiant, this is time for 'pack your shit and go' therapy."[8] This is when "cutting him off" means exactly that: cutting off all sources of enablement—financial, housing, employment, all services, and any other means of support.

If the victim is living at home, she has to leave the house immediately—not tomorrow, not next week. Now. If she lives outside the family home and you, the parents, are paying her rent and utilities or supplementing her income in other ways, that ends right now. She can sleep on friends' couches until they tire of her mooching. You must take away the car, but if it is in her name, you must stop the car payments and stop paying for insurance, gas, and maintenance.

Same goes with the cell phone. She'll have to figure out a way to pay for it. In other words, she's really on her own—unless she accepts their gift and goes to rehab.

Here's where parents usually ask themselves, "What kind of parents are we? Who could do this to their own flesh and blood?" A parent who wants to save their child, that's who. That applies to other family members as well. All it takes is one relative or friend to feel sorry for the victim, and the enablement continues. Otherwise, that is the only way this works.

If the individual surrenders, it doesn't necessarily happen within the allotted hour of a television program. Depending on the leverage, surrender could take minutes, hours, days, weeks, or months. I've experienced them all. Since a bed is not always available when the client is, it is also essential that, prior to the intervention, one or more alternate facilities have been chosen and are ready for the individual's arrival as well.

Joseph and Betty of Minneapolis are the parents of a son, Barry, whose failure to launch rendered him an unemployed thirty-something man hopelessly and chronically addicted to meth. The only leverage they had was evicting him from one of their rental properties where he had been living rent free. I warned them that getting Barry to treatment could take six minutes, six hours, six days, six weeks, or six months—or it might not happen at all. Despite the hard-core stance they had to maintain, Joe and Betty were in—committed. They knew nothing else was going to work.

It took six weeks of no utilities and finally a sheriff's order to evict Barry. Then homeless, he eventually saw the wisdom of surrendering and accepted his parents' gift of treatment. Upon Barry's admission to Casa Colina in Texas, Joe and Betty saw the detritus of their son's addiction when they inspected the rental house. Every appliance, copper pipe, and wire had been ripped out and sold to support his destructive habit.

During this six-week odyssey from hell, Barry hated me with a vengeance and treated me so. Understandably, since I was his addiction's enemy, and it did everything to fight me. On day 45 of his ninety days of formal treatment, I got a call. "Walter, this is Barry. I want you to know that I love you . . . you saved my life."

Again, that's something one doesn't hear every day, and I appreciate it when I do. But in reality, it's Barry and his parents who deserve the accolades. It was their fortitude and Barry's eventual wisdom that were responsible for his recovery.

If the individual is totally dependent on the family or one source, the leverage is concentrated and easy to apply, and it usually results in surrender—immediately or eventually. However, the more diverse the enablement, the thinner the leverage over the victim. Generally, the more functional and independent the individual is—for example, if he is employed, the beneficiary of a trust fund, or a successful business owner who lives outside of the family home and provides for himself—the weaker the leverage a family or loved ones can apply on that individual. It usually comes down to emotional leverage at that point, which is exceedingly difficult to pull off. His addiction couldn't give a shit how you feel.

In most cases, however, the addiction and problems that come with it—car accidents, physical injury, health problems, arrests, incarceration, legal fees, accidental overdose, loss of employment, and loss of friends and family, among other things—consume most, if not all, of the individual's resources. At that point, most of the time the individual sees the inevitable and is forced to surrender—or sometimes doesn't. Tragically, not all endings are happy.

Then there are instances when the individual is in major crisis and needs stabilization before addiction treatment can even be discussed.

I got a call from a panicked Sharon, who was on her way to my office with her adult nephew, Jake. Although previously compliant, Jake popped out of the car at an intersection to launch into a meth-induced rant threatening terrified commuters waiting for the light to change. Sharon, overcome with fear, screamed over the phone for help. I told her to lock her doors while I called 911 and insisted that an officer from the city's crisis intervention team accompany the responding officers. Within twenty minutes, a restrained Jake was in the back seat of a patrol car on the way to the city's crisis intervention center.

Two days later, for our initial meeting, I visited Jake at the center. Although it had been forty-eight hours, he was still in an agitated state and particularly angry at me. After three minutes, knowing that this meeting was not going to end well, I got up to leave, and that's when he lunged at me from across the table, screaming at the top of his lungs. That's precisely when I realized why the three-hundred-pound tech was sitting at the back of the room this whole time. It was only nanoseconds before a stream of other techs magically appeared to join him in restraining Jake while ordering me out of the room.

A word of caution here: If the individual is experiencing what health care professionals call a "psychotic break"—such as admitting to having suicide ideation, verbally threatening to commit suicide, threatening to harm a third party—or you just feel he's capable of doing something drastic, call 911 or immediately take or get that person to a crisis intervention center, acute psychiatric unit, or emergency room right away. Take no chances. After stabilization, the individual can be assessed later for long-term treatment.

By the way, although it was a tortuous year getting him to treatment, Jake's journey through two rehabs in southern California led him to his dream job—working at a golf course in Arizona.

CHAPTER FIVE

THE RIGHT PLAN

"Because drug addiction is typically a chronic disorder character-ized by occasional relapses, a short-term, one-time treatment is usually not sufficient. For many, treatment is a long-term process that involves multiple interventions and regular monitoring."[1]

"So today, start where you are—not where you wish you were, but where you are."

—Maria Shriver[2]

Structure of the Right Plan

Like other chronic diseases, addiction can be managed through the right treatment, lifelong mutual support, and a self-management system that fits the individual and her resources.

There is no one plan that fits everyone. Does each plan always follow the script? When you have human beings and a relentless disease involved, don't count on it. Will there be changes along the way? Of course—name me one chronic disease where treatment goes exactly as initially planned.

Will there be setbacks? Hope there aren't, but plan there will be. The chronic nature of addiction means that relapsing is not only

Comparison of relapse rates between drug addiction and other chronic illnesses

Percentage of patients who relapse

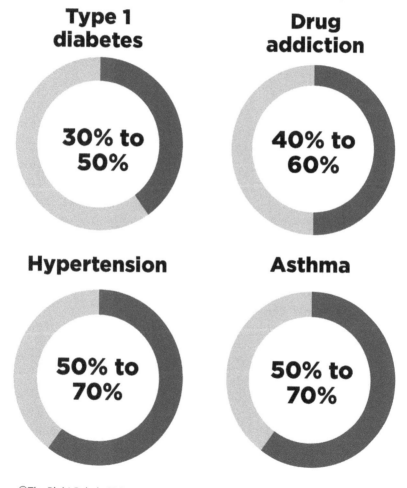

Type 1 diabetes
30% to 50%

Drug addiction
40% to 60%

Hypertension
50% to 70%

Asthma
50% to 70%

©The Right Rehab, LLC

Figure 5.1.

Source: National Institute on Drug Abuse, "What Is Drug Addiction Treatment?" (2020). Art © The Right Rehab, LLC.

possible but also likely since its recurrence rates are similar to other chronic diseases (see figure 5.1).

"Key components of care are medications, behavioral therapies and recovery support services (RSS)."

—Vivek H. Murthy (MD, MBA),
U.S. surgeon general, 2014–2017, 2021–[3]

According to the National Institute on Drug Abuse (NIDA), the best way to prevent relapse is structuring the right plan for the individual, knowing that it will need adjustments along the way (see figure 5.2). A person in treatment may require varying combinations of services during its course, including ongoing assessment. "For most people, a continuing care approach provides the best results, with each treatment level adapted to a person's changing needs."[4]

Research studies confirm and treatment experts insist that anything less than ninety days of formal treatment, including medications and behavioral therapies, is of limited effectiveness. If one has the resources, there are facilities with even longer programs of six months, nine months, or one year. Whatever the plan, the right one for the right someone is supported by a foundation of the following five components (see figure 5.3):

1. Diagnosis
2. Resources
3. A customized treatment plan that fits the individual and resources
4. Adjustments when necessary
5. Commitment to making it work

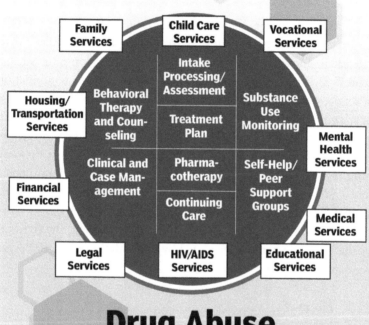

Components of Comprehensive

Family Services

Child Care Services

Vocational Services

Housing/Transportation Services

Behavioral Therapy and Counseling

Intake Processing/Assessment

Treatment Plan

Substance Use Monitoring

Mental Health Services

Financial Services

Clinical and Case Management

Pharmacotherapy

Continuing Care

Self-Help/Peer Support Groups

Medical Services

Legal Services

HIV/AIDS Services

Educational Services

Drug Abuse Treatment

The best treatment programs provide a combination of therapies and other services to meet the needs of the individual patient.

©The Right Rehab, LLC

Figure 5.2.

Source: National Institute on Drug Abuse, "How Effective Is Drug Abuse Treatment?" (2018). Art © The Right Rehab, LLC.

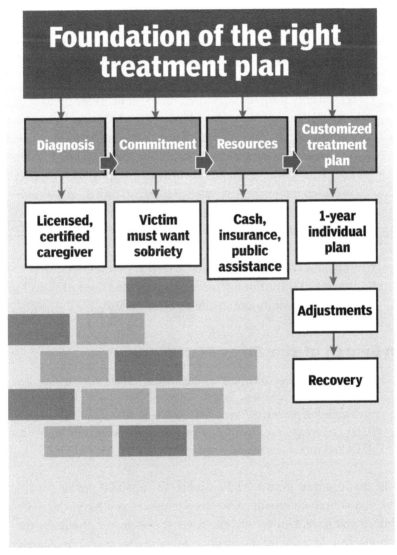

Figure 5.3.
Art © The Right Rehab, LLC.

Based on that foundation, a customized treatment plan is structured upon the following common denominators:

- Treatment has to be tailored to each person's diagnosis; drug-use patterns; drug-related medical, mental, and social issues; and resources.
- If resources allow, a customized one-year plan (see figure 5.4) should be ninety days of evidence-based behavioral therapy, medication, and transitional living followed by an ongoing continuum of care plan of recovery support services (RSS).
- The RSS must include sober living, mutual-aid support (meetings), new positive relationships, and work or continuing education in an environment supportive of a recovery lifestyle that becomes a road map for a lifetime of continued recovery.
- Individual and group outpatient sessions during aftercare.
- If necessary, continuing medication-assisted therapy (MAT) but with a plan to eventually taper off its use.

In Search of the Right Plan

Recovery: A process of change through which individuals improve their health and wellness, live self-directed lives, and strive to reach their full potential. Even individuals with severe and chronic SUDs [substance use disorders] can, with help, overcome their SUDs and regain health and social function.[5]

Treatment ranges from a Malibu rehab for $240,000 to one that's free in a church basement. The more resources you have, the more options you have. Conversely, the fewer the resources, the fewer the options. But do more resources alone guarantee recovery? Absolutely not. Whether it's at a recovery version of Club Med or a puke-green-painted basement with folding chairs, recovery is ultimately up to the individual no matter where it occurs.

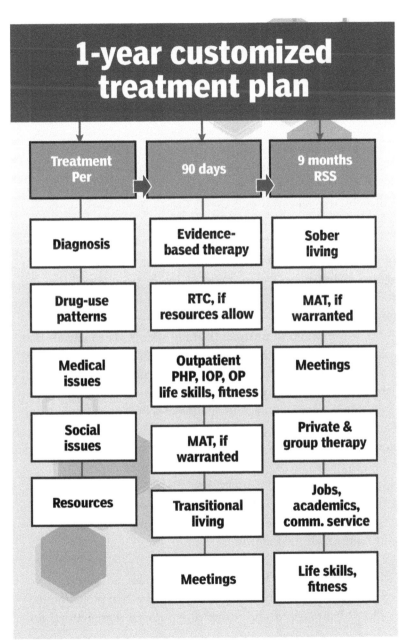

Figure 5.4.
Art © The Right Rehab, LLC.

"I call it 'spontaneous remission,' and whether it happens with no warning or after an avalanche of consequences, what matters is that it happens and you hold on to it."

—William Cope Moyers[6]

Rachel Miller of the nationwide treatment provider Summit Behavioral Health is a living, breathing example of just that: "I didn't even know that treatment was an option. I simply walked into an AA meeting knowing I had to change my life. That community of strangers who told me to keep coming back supported me on my journey and made me the person who I am today. No one—most of all myself—could have predicted my life today. I am five years sober and proud to work for one of the country's largest treatment companies. I am grateful for all the pain, grateful for the struggle, grateful for my sobriety because I would not be the person who I am today."[7]

So, why even go to treatment? Study after study concludes that the longer one's formal treatment, the better the results in achieving sobriety and living a true recovery lifestyle: ninety days of formal treatment at a specialty facility—including residential treatment—followed by a minimum of nine months of sober living (three years, ideally), mutual support group(s) (Alcoholics Anonymous, Narcotics Anonymous, SMART Recovery, etc.), and MAT (if necessary). According to treatment professionals with decades of experience in the field, these steps, combined with several other customized factors, are the optimum ways to attain and sustain a recovery lifestyle.

A conventional ninety-day plan (see figure 5.5) at a specialty facility consists of the following:

Days 1 through 30: RTC* (residential treatment center)
Days 31 through 60: PHP (partial hospitalization programming)
Days 61 through 90: IOP (intensive outpatient programming)

---

*Different rehabs have different policies regarding whether detox days should be counted as residential days.

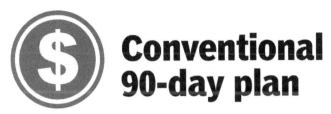

Conventional 90-day plan

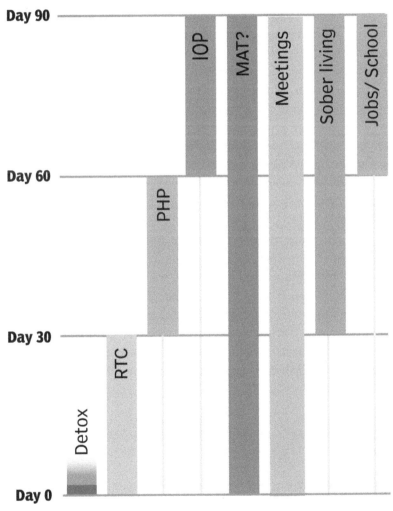

©The Right Rehab, LLC

Figure 5.5.
Art © The Right Rehab, LLC.

As it is with most things in life, the kind of treatment one gets usually comes down to one common denominator: resources. These days, the best way to ensure a full ninety days of specialty treatment is "private pay"—in other words, cash. What one can afford usually determines the kind of treatment one gets.

The good news about private pay is that I can't think of any rehab that won't take your money. Most facilities will work with you on a payment schedule; the facility has inherent control to customize and execute the number of days one is in a particular treatment regimen; and depending on the facility, you can get a lot of bells and whistles that will make you feel, "Hey, rehab isn't so bad. I can do this."

The bad news is that not everyone can afford anywhere from $15,000 to $80,000 per month for treatment. Also, maybe it's just me, but in my experience with clients, turning addiction treatment into a Club Med experience (minus the alcohol, of course) does not necessarily induce deep introspection and help in answering "Why am I so fucked up?"

Does the more money you pay for treatment guarantee long-term sobriety? No. Many individuals in recovery didn't go to rehab at all—twelve-step meetings are their therapy.

The point is that what works for one person does not mean it will work for another. One person's remission, recovery, and long-term recovery is completely up to that individual, no matter the number of treatments and the sums of money spent. Resources help equip the individual with more tools, but the question always comes down to this: "Does the individual *really* want to get and stay sober?

Insurance—It's Not Always What You Think It Is

"But I have insurance, why do I need to pay anything?" is a refrain I hear constantly. It's surprising how many people don't realize that an insurance policy doesn't mean you don't have to spend cash; sometimes you must spend a great deal of it. And on top of that, some carriers don't allow for residential treatment, especially some policies for state and county employees, as well as Medicare and Medicaid in several states throughout the nation.

Historically, private health insurance has been responsible for countless people getting the substance use disorder (SUD) or mental health treatment they sorely needed and otherwise would have never received. Hands down, it has saved lives. Period.

Unfortunately, that's changed.

Today, the increase in the number of people who need treatment and the general escalation of health care costs have completely changed the economics and structure of substance use disorder treatment. Just because one may have an insurance policy with one of the long-established insurance companies—Blue Cross, Aetna, United Healthcare, Cigna, for example—there are still premiums, co-payments, deductibles, out-of-pocket maximums, and upfront payments.

Today, I see scores of people who take out policies just so they can have one in case of catastrophic illness, but these policies come with deductibles and out-of-pocket maximums that are out of reach. If you can't afford an upfront payment for your unmet deductible and out-of-pocket maximum—say, between $2,500 and $15,000—plus the room and board costs that are *not* covered by insurance, your insurance policy for behavioral health isn't a big help.

In the first half of 2020, 43.4 percent of adults (97.8 million) were inadequately insured. And just because you are one of the lucky ones to have health insurance through your employer, guess what? One-quarter of the 122 million of you (30.5 million) were underinsured. In fact, employer-provided insurance has the highest rate of those who are underinsured because larger portions of the premiums are being carried by the employee and deductibles and out-of-pocket maximums are rising at rates much higher than employee compensation.[8] Every day, scores of people are discovering that, even with their health insurance policy, they still can't afford treatment.

Nowadays, getting ninety days of treatment at a specialty facility—including residential—solely through one's insurance policy is pretty much a pipedream. Nonetheless, if one has access to supplemental cash, it can be used to one's advantage by dramatically contributing to treatment at a facility that otherwise would not be affordable.

In any event, it is necessary to know which payment options are accepted at facilities (see figure 5.6).

Treatment is mostly covered by a combination of several sources such as private health insurance + private pay, Medicaid + other public assistance, or cash for residential treatment + insurance that only covers outpatient programming.

In describing the right plan, let's design a one-year treatment plan—private pay and/or private health insurance—to start with ninety days of treatment at a specialty facility that includes residential treatment. Some specialty facilities' ninety-day programs house the patients entirely in one setting, while others institute off-site outpatient programming combined with off-site sober living after the initial residential stage of treatment.

Diagnosis

> "In order to design a plan, one must know the diagnosis."
>
> —Walter Wolf

Once there is a diagnosis, the facilities specializing in that particular diagnosis are immediately options for a client's placement. Treatment facilities need to be licensed by the state in which they practice, therefore, knowing a facility's licensure is key when determining the ones to be considered candidates for a client's treatment. Licensure normally falls into one of five categories:

1. Substance abuse
2. Mental health
3. Primary substance abuse, secondary mental health
4. Primary mental health, secondary substance abuse
5. Primary mental disorder and primary substance abuse

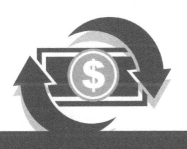

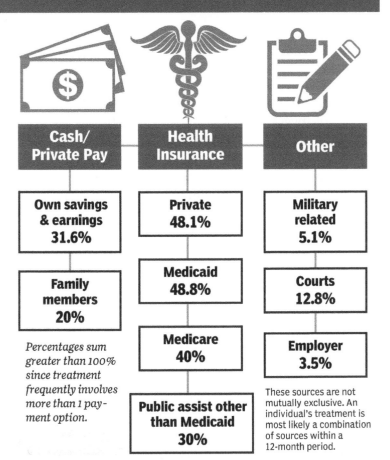

Cash/ Private Pay	Health Insurance	Other
Own savings & earnings 31.6%	Private 48.1%	Military related 5.1%
Family members 20%	Medicaid 48.8%	Courts 12.8%
Percentages sum greater than 100% since treatment frequently involves more than 1 payment option.	Medicare 40%	Employer 3.5%
	Public assist other than Medicaid 30%	These sources are not mutually exclusive. An individual's treatment is most likely a combination of sources within a 12-month period.

Figure 5.6. 2019 Source of Payment

Source: Center for Behavioral Health Statistics and Quality (2020). Art © The Right Rehab, LLC.

It's easy to get lost in the weeds when it comes to these details, but it is these details that determine which facilities are positioned to deliver the best treatment per diagnosis. For myself, numerous details—including the treatment staff, their accessibility, executive leadership, strengths of their program, and their past care of my clients—play a huge role. There are treatment programs that specialize in different diagnoses—the key is knowing who they are and whether they deliver what they promise.

Location

Location of the rehab should not be local nor relatively close to home—especially for a millennial. Avoid one that is an easy exit out the door, close to the world and people from which he is escaping—the "land of triggers." A "trigger" is anything that makes a person crave a drug or alcohol—sounds, odors, people, and locations from drug-using days, for example—sometimes without even the individual being consciously aware of the triggering event.

If the individual is away in an unfamiliar location, it's easier to avoid those environmental cues. It has to be far enough away—not on the other side of the door—where a call to a friend for a ride or an easy hitch-hike down the interstate can't fix a craving. Especially if the individual is experiencing withdrawal, it's tempting to exit the facility to quickly fix the pain.

I learned this truth firsthand when taking a heroin-addicted client to detox on the south side of town. I should have known there would be a problem when, as we entered the hospital, he stopped, took in the neighborhood, and remarked, "Funny, this is where I buy my drugs." I no longer take clients there for detox.

The individual leaving the facility against medical advice—AMA—is something to avoid at all costs. However, as long as the patient is an adult, she is free to leave the facility anytime, despite the facility's best efforts to persuade her that leaving early is against her own best interests. An individual can be held against her own will in a "lockdown" crisis intervention facility if she is a danger to herself or someone else—usually only for a seventy-two-hour period (but longer if the acuity is high enough).

Otherwise, it is illegal to hold an individual against his will without an emergency court order or unless you are in a state whose justice system has a process that allows long-term involuntary detainment, such as Florida. Florida has two laws—the Baker Act and the Marchman Act—on its books that have become indispensable for the safety of those who have been threatened by individuals who have demonstrated to be a plausible danger to others.

In the United States, it is not against the law to be crazy. It is against the law to be a danger to someone else. When families ask me to send their loved one to a facility where the individual can't just walk out, I explain that it's not possible under most circumstances. The loved one must realize that he needs to be there and that walking out is a choice that is not right for him.

Paul's mother called me in a panic. The Pittsburgh police had just raided her twenty-five-year-old son's home and had him in custody for placing threatening calls to police departments throughout the country. While in custody, his interrogation revealed that Paul was not the danger; his mental illness was the culprit. He needed help they couldn't provide. When I arrived in Pittsburgh, Paul was already in the local crisis intervention center with a classic dual diagnosis of paranoid schizophrenia with accompanying meth abuse. With the help of an off-duty cop and medication for the flight, I escorted Paul across the country to a long-term program at the primary mental health, secondary substance abuse facility that best fit him. While there, on several occasions Paul threatened to flee the facility. The staff told him he could walk out the front door anytime, but it really was not a good idea.

Paul stayed for eight months. Eight months. How is that? Paul could have walked out anytime but figured out that he needed to be there and took advantage of their care. Today, he is working at the very crisis intervention center that held him back in Pittsburgh.

The takeaway is this: There are both excellent and harmful treatment programs and facilities throughout the country. The key is knowing how to determine the *right one* for a particular, singular individual and diagnosis.

There are also ways to make an early exit an inconvenient—if not difficult—task. That includes limiting the funds available to the individual—no credit cards and little to no cash—which will make transportation or lodging unlikely without direct help from a third party. Minimal funds should be available to the individual on a weekly basis through the facility or a debit card for occasional group trips off campus for meals, toiletries, movies, and such, but that's all. The rehab will tell you how much to send. Walking out the door into a location with no contacts, no cash, and no credit cards makes an early exit less enticing.

A totally new environment offers another critical component in the individual's treatment—there's an opportunity to leave the previous life of addiction and addiction-related relationships physically behind. It will give the individual time to start a new life with others in similar circumstances and become part of a community supporting each other in sobriety and working toward a life of recovery.

I tell parents that the phone call they want from their child after forty-five or fifty days is "I'm not coming home." What she's saying is that she's found a new life, one of sobriety and recovery. Her friends and relationships—her whole environment—are no longer centered on drugs and their destructive habits. Now she has the support to build a new, sober life. That's not impossible in her previous life's environment, but starting over in a different location brings advantages her previous home will never have.

Good examples of locations where a millennial can easily start a new life with world-class rehabs, reliable aftercare, a supportive sober community, and several educational institutions include Lubbock, Texas; Nashville, Tennessee; Dallas, Texas; Newport Beach, California; Atlanta, Georgia; and Austin, Texas—just to name a few.

Of course, when it comes to a head of family or an adult with a job and family responsibilities, going away for ninety days, much less one year, most often is not a viable option. However, going away for at least the first thirty days, then following with a continuum of care using local resources for sixty days of PHP and IOP services, is a definite option for following a ninety-day formal treatment plan.

For employees whose employer is an active supporter of one's treatment, keeping one's job open usually entails a regimen of random drug testing, regular attendance at twelve-step meetings, and performance reviews upon return. An employee who receives the active support of the employer during treatment and recovery most often turn out to be that employer's most productive and loyal worker.

Intake

If the physical and behavioral condition of the patient requires immediate medical attention, one of the following must occur:

- Admission to a detoxification unit for managed substance withdrawal
- General hospital admission for addiction-related medical ailments
- Admission to an acute unit for behavioral stabilization

Those conditions take priority. The following assessment process would take place after the patient is stabilized.

Although the individual is assessed by a facility clinician over the phone prior to travel, a more detailed clinical assessment by a licensed drug and alcohol counselor, psychiatrist, or psychologist, plus a physical exam by a physician, occurs upon arrival at the facility. This intake process includes a screening for substances, a detailed history of abusing them, a mental health evaluation, and a contraband/prohibited items check of the individual's personal items. Plan on this process taking several hours. See figure 5.7.

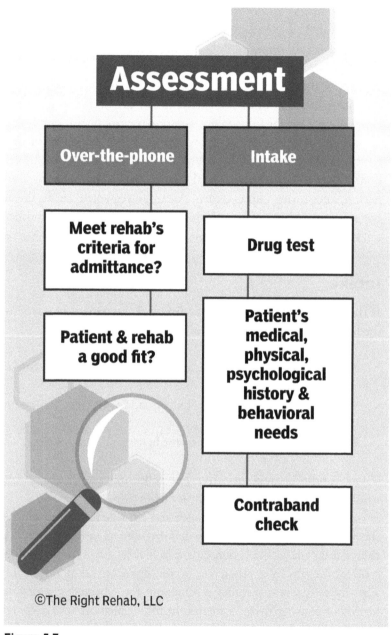

Figure 5.7.
Art © The Right Rehab, LLC.

This assessment is necessary for understanding the nature and severity of the individual's health, social, and familial problems that led to the current situation. Those issues include the following:

- Age, gender, and ethnicity
- Substance(s) of choice, length of use, and date and amount last used
- Current health issues or needs
- Medical history
- Family history of substance use and mental disorders
- Suicide attempts or ideation
- Current medications
- Effects of substances on the person's life
- Cultural issues around the use of alcohol or drugs
- Familial relationships
- Social relationships, issues, and needs
- Legal or financial problems
- Current living situation
- Employment history, stability, problems, and needs
- If relevant, school performance, problems, and needs
- Any previous treatment experiences or attempts to stop substance use
- The patient's desires for his life

Understanding each person's unique physical, psychological, and behavioral needs—plus the intensity and nature of their SUD—leads to outlining a year-long treatment plan that determines the intensity and composition of the first ninety days of formal treatment followed by an aftercare program. As a person's lifetime hopefully is a long one, the plan must be continually assessed and modified to meet the individual's changing needs.

As previously mentioned, during this assessment it is imperative that the patient be completely honest with his answers, especially if the treatment is insurance dependent. If the individual needs insurance to cover treatment, the results of the exam are immediately relayed to the insurance company for their required authorization to start treatment. As long as the results of the assessment fit their criteria for "medical necessity"—presence of drugs or alcohol in the system or the patient's drug history, for example—they will authorize treatment, at least for the first stage of treatment, which is usually (but not always) detox, followed by residential treatment. If the appropriate level of substances is not present, the insurance company does not consider that person "acute" or the requested level of care— detox and/or residential—"medically necessary."

And here is the brutal catch-22 when it comes to treatment and the insurance company: It's natural to think that if you are suffering from substance addiction and you've managed not to have "used" for several days before you go to treatment, that's a good thing, right? Not so fast.

There's an unwritten rule when determining the level of treatment that the insurance company will authorize upon entering drug and alcohol treatment. Prior to arrival, rehabs say that if the person has not used within the past five days, the insurance company most likely will determine that the level of substances in the system are *not* high enough to justify detox and residential treatment. This is possibly the same for the next level of care—partial hospitalization programming (PHP)—as well. That leaves the next two levels— intensive outpatient programming (IOP) and outpatient programming (OP)—which are both considerably less intensive, much thinner treatments normally for those who have already been through detox, residential, and PHP. Most important to the insurance company, IOP and OP are much less expensive treatment levels for them to reimburse the facility. It's as if the individual's previous years of heavy abuse never happened.

So, here's the really sick part regarding most insurance coverage: to get treatment for a life of getting loaded, you have to be loaded. Although they won't explicitly tell you to use before you get to them, that's exactly what rehabs mean when they say, "Don't change your behavior prior to coming to us." In other words, have shit in your system when you arrive.

Need another reason to get the individual to treatment as soon as possible? Now you know.

Detox

Detox (detoxification) is medically supervised withdrawal and stabilization in an inpatient hospital or hospital-type setting with twenty-four-hour hospital-type care. At best stabilization, the purpose is to make a patient medically stable and as free as possible of substances prior to long-term treatment, with typically thirty days of residential treatment as the next stage. Many facilities place the client in detox for the first twenty-four hours for observation as a matter of course anyway. Units set up specifically for detox are located in hospitals, rehab facilities, or third-party independent units. Detox consists of three components (see figure 5.8):

- Evaluation regarding whether the substances ingested require medically assisted withdrawal. If needed, it could last three to ten days, depending upon the substance(s) involved.
- Stabilization. Alcohol, opioid, and tranquilizer abuse produces significant physical withdrawal side effects that can lead to seizures and other health consequences. Their misuse requires withdrawal management for sometimes up to ten days.

  Marijuana, stimulants, and meth typically produce primarily emotional and cognitive symptoms, which do not automatically require physical withdrawal management. However, people who abuse stimulants usually become addicted to other substances (such as alcohol, sedatives, or opioids) and, therefore, can experience any of the complications ascribed to detoxification from these substances. An often overlooked, but potentially lethal, medical danger during stimulant withdrawal is the risk of a profound

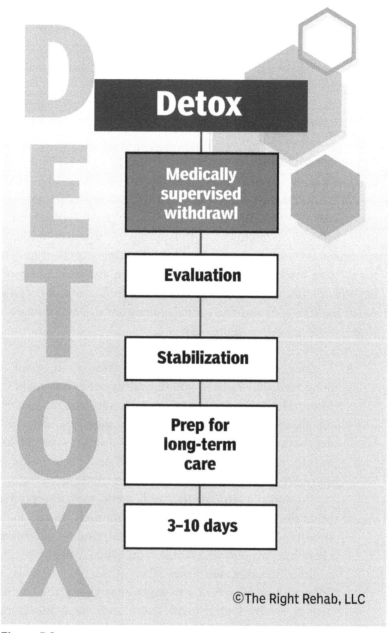

Figure 5.8.
Art © The Right Rehab, LLC.

dysphoria—depression, negative thoughts and feelings—that may include suicidal ideation or attempts.

Since the period of depression experienced by amphetamine users is more prolonged and may be more intense, the patient should be monitored closely during detoxification for signs of suicidality and treated for depression if appropriate. Patients with recent cocaine use can experience cardiac problems, including heart attack.[9]

- Preparation for long-term care, such as residential treatment, which is the next step of a one-year treatment plan. Considered the first step in SUD treatment, detox is stabilization at best, but it is not an effective treatment for SUDs. Studies have found that half to three-quarters of individuals with SUDs who receive withdrawal management services do not enter treatment on their own accord.[10]

At several rehabs, the patient is automatically placed in the detox unit for twenty-four hours of observation to determine whether the person is facing withdrawal. It is also an early warning sign regarding whether the individual is committed to getting sober. As already mentioned in chapter 3, it is not uncommon for a victim to go through detox and mistake being "clean" for being "cured" and, therefore, believe that further treatment is no longer required. This is an extremely bad development since the patient is in increased danger of death by overdose, as her tolerance to the substance she was previously ingesting is now drastically reduced.

Jimmy worked on an oil rig in North Dakota. He picked up a heroin addiction—like his fellow crew mates—due to the crushing boredom they endured during their time off up there. Since he promised his young wife—his third marriage at thirty-four years old—that he would get straight, he came to me for placement in a ninety-day treatment program. Upon arrival in detox, Jimmy announced to the staff that he was going to be "cured" in four days. That would be a first, but the staff was always up for something new. On the morning of day 5, Jimmy left the rehab against medical advice and checked into a motel. No one has heard from him since.

Under private pay, I've seen detox units charge anywhere from $500 to $2,250 per day. Typically the most expensive stage of treatment, detox is ironically one stage of treatment where I have seen all different kinds of insurance companies cover without too much pushback.

Residential Treatment Center (RTC)

Residential treatment, or RTC (short for "residential treatment center"), typically takes place in a hospital-like setting for a twenty-four-hour, thirty-day highly structured and supervised program using evidence-based therapies, medication, and clinical and holistic services. The facility also provides living quarters for the patients, hence "residential." Its setting can be rural or urban, on a campus in a dormitory-like setting, in cottages, or in residential home or apartment where all associated activities take place. See figure 5.9.

The real meat and potatoes of treatment, residential care focuses on modifying behavior regarding substance use, resocializing individuals through personal accountability and responsibility, and helping people build socially productive lives. The program's highly structured treatment can be confrontational with activities designed to help residents examine damaging beliefs, self-concepts, and destructive patterns of behavior and adopt new, more harmonious, and constructive ways to interact with others. It's a stage when a palette of services that meet specific medical, mental, social, occupational, family, and legal needs of the individual is used to address the needs of the whole person in order to be successful.[11]

Residential treatment is the stage when attendance at twelve-step meetings or alternative support groups becomes a fixture in the recovering victim's life. Meetings occur on-site, but most facilities also take residents to meetings off-site several times a week, which is an important opportunity for the individual to be a member of a

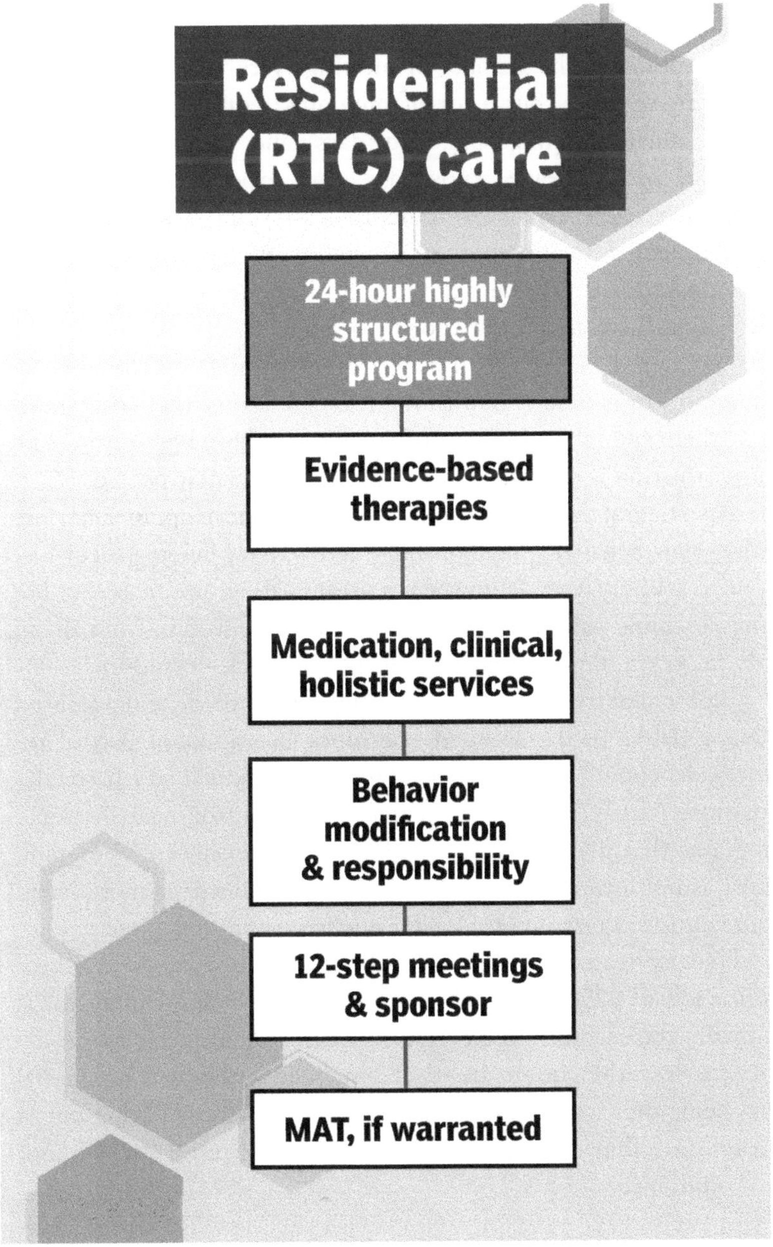

Residential (RTC) care

- 24-hour highly structured program
- Evidence-based therapies
- Medication, clinical, holistic services
- Behavior modification & responsibility
- 12-step meetings & sponsor
- MAT, if warranted

Figure 5.9.
Art © The Right Rehab, LLC.

wider community and start creating a new social network of those also in sobriety. The number of meetings vary with the particular treatment regimen, but a lot of programs require participants to attend "ninety meetings in ninety days" and to get a sponsor—someone with mileage, knowledge, and experience the newbie doesn't have—an "Obi-Wan Kenobi" to the young initiate.

Residential treatment is a fascinating metamorphosis as the individual realizes that he is not the only one confronting similar issues—that there are others who are in more or less dire situations. I have witnessed those in total denial prior to admission who, by day 30, are converts when hit with the realization that they really need to be there and take advantage of the gift they have been given. The transformation is stunning; they literally become new people.

An integral part of the transformation is developing sober life skills—new behaviors, relationships, and ways of living a sober life. Prior to sobriety, the victim spent a great deal—if not most—of her time obtaining substances, using them, and recovering from them, only to obtain more substances and start the cycle over again.

Residential treatment is also the stage when medication-assisted therapy (MAT)—if warranted—becomes an important part of recovery depending upon the facility and the individual's particular situation. MAT is relatively new and still controversial for some programs that maintain a conventional "abstinence only" program. MAT is not meant to be used by itself, as its effectiveness is linked with continued use of behavioral, evidence-based therapies.

Under private pay, I've seen residential treatment run anywhere from a low of $250 to as high as $2,666 per day. Residential care is normally the second-most expensive of treatment levels for insurance carriers; the current trend of insurance-authorized residential days being drastically reduced does not apply to those paying out of pocket since they can receive a full thirty days of residential without interruption (figure 5.10).

The surest way to get 30 days of RTC is with Private Pay.

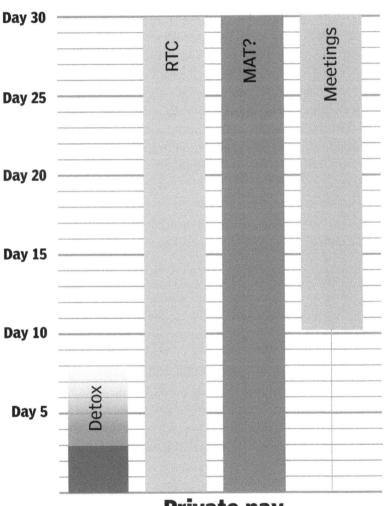

Figure 5.10.
Art © The Right Rehab, LLC.

Another Word about Insurance

Under private health insurance, how many days of residential care will an insurance company cover? No telling. The rehab can't guarantee that number, although there are rare instances when a rehab will squeeze twenty-eight or thirty days of RTC coverage. The only real evidence I have is the number of days a particular insurance company has been recently authorizing, which is almost never thirty days for RTC these days, but I am shocked by the rare occasion when a client of mine will get forty-eight days of authorized RTC. When that happens, it's usually with a regional insurance company that has a long-established history with a particular facility.

Whenever I have a client using insurance for treatment, I send the individual's insurance information (usually a picture of the front and back of the insurance card) right away to the rehab for a VOB (verification of benefits). The rehab comes back with the following:

- The deductible and maximum out-of-pocket amounts still unmet
- The co-pay schedules
- Status of premiums paid
- Any special notes from the insurance carrier
- The upfront amount payable to the rehab
- Appropriateness of the rehab/patient match

The total of the unmet deductible and maximum out of pocket is important since facilities typically need that amount upfront, upon admission. Then I need an estimate or at least a range of the number of days my client can expect the insurance company to cover for each level of treatment. As already stated, the rehab cannot guarantee the number of days the insurance carrier will authorize.

It is the rehab's job to treat the patient while updating the carrier on the patient's vitals and the medical necessity for further treatment. It's the insurance carrier that needs to be convinced of the continued medical necessity for each level of treatment—not the facility.

When I started working with families, one phone call from the rehab for authorization of twenty-eight to thirty days of residential treatment from the insurance carrier was most often the case. These days, there has been a rapid decline of days authorized, especially for residential treatment. What used to be automatically twenty-eight authorized days of residential treatment is now between fourteen and twenty-five days—and even as few as six days (including detox). And to get that authorization, what used to be one call from the rehab is now a call every three, five, seven, or ten days to the carrier to authorize treatment for those many more days at a time (figure 5.11).

Most insurance companies will at least give a heads-up to a facility when a patient's level of treatment is about to change. There are outliers, however. One admissions person at a rehab where I know my clients always get optimum care can't stand doing business with a huge and well-known insurance carrier's policies out of Florida and Texas. Instead of the insurance carrier warning that they are stepping down a patient's level of care on a certain date, they just go ahead and do it. There are even instances when the insurance carrier will pull a patient's care altogether. No warning. Just "Send the guy home."

Imagine taking your car to the mechanic. It's got all kinds of problems. It needs a new transmission, carburetor, radiator, and steering wheel. A few days later, you go to pick it up and it runs great; the engine has never run better, and the mechanic did a fabulous job. But where's the steering wheel? You can't drive the car without it. The mechanic says he repeatedly told that to the insurance company, but they insisted, "We spent enough money on the engine; the rest is up to him."

Is that experience universal and happening at all rehabs that take insurance? I wish I could say no, but nowadays that's pretty much the norm.

There are several variables at play here—the state where a rehab is located, the state from which the insurance is issued, the individual's benefits, and the relationship between the facility and the insurance carrier. For instance, there are a few facilities that guarantee twenty-

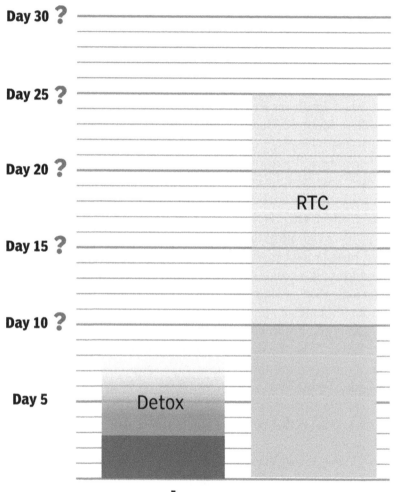

Figure 5.11.
Art © The Right Rehab, LLC.

eight days of residential treatment because of a special contract they have with an insurance company, such as Caron's women's trauma treatment program and Blue Cross Blue Shield. Blue Cross Federal will also frequently be more liberal authorizing residential days at certain facilities. But, at the majority of facilities, those examples are rare to nonexistent.

Frequently, a number of days will be quoted at one facility, but a totally different number will be quoted at another one located in a different state. It's the same policy, same individual, and same diagnosis, but there's a completely different number of days likely to be authorized.

Don't think this is the fault of the rehab, because it's not. The most expensive levels of treatment in descending order are detox, residential, PHP, IOP, and OP. The lower the level of treatment is, the less money the insurance company has to reimburse the facility. This explains the insurance company's desire to step the client down to a lower level of care at the soonest date.

Since they control the purse strings, today it's the insurance companies that have the last say regarding which levels of care meet the medical necessity for a particular patient. Those decisions are made by a physician working for the insurance company who has never met the patient, most likely has never visited the rehab, and quite possibly has limited or no experience with addiction treatment prior to this assignment. But that physician has final say over what kind of treatment that patient needs at that particular moment.

On those occasions when the rehab and the insurance company disagree on stepping a patient down to a lower level of care, the rehab's attending physician can appeal the decision to the physician working for the insurance company, which is called a "peer-to-peer" conference or review. More often than not, the insurance company's decision is upheld, despite what the physician on scene has to say. Comforting, right?

Now, why is it a big deal that the number of days the insurance company will authorize for residential treatment reduces from twenty-eight or thirty days to now fewer (and sometimes as low as six days)? At most rehabs (not all, but most of them), on the first day of the lower level of care—usually to PHP from residential—the billing is bifurcated.

In most cases, nothing changes as far as the patient is concerned—he will still sleep in the same bed and continue his current programming until day 30. Insurance will continue reimbursing the rehab for treatment (albeit now at a lower rate), but most—not all—rehabs now will charge the patient for room and board. In effect, the rehab is still providing the same level of care but at a lower reimbursement rate from the insurance company. Some rehabs are constrained by state laws that prohibit an insurance company's reimbursement being used for anything other than treatment. Room and board are not considered treatment. In some states—California, for instance—by law, the patient's housing must change from the residential setting to a separate sober living environment when the patient is stepped down to PHP.

I have seen a range of $25–$300 per day for room and board. Some rehabs will charge in arrears, but some will ask for a two-week deposit upon admission.

For some clients who need their insurance policy to get treatment, coming up with a $780–$3,000 deposit for two weeks of room and board is a deal killer. It doesn't end there. Some facilities have to ask for an additional deposit, sometimes as much as $10,000, to guard against the insurance company suddenly pulling all further coverage for a particular patient's stay.

For those reasons, I always ask for the most recent history of the number of days the insurance company has been authorizing for all levels of treatment—residential, PHP, and IOP. I know that the rehab cannot guarantee the number of days the insurance company will cover—that is out of their control—but it's my job to tell the patient's financial guarantor what to expect regarding costs (remember, no surprises).

Thirty-two-year-old James's diagnosis was primary mental disorder (bipolar and mild personality disorder) with secondary substance abuse (chronic meth use). James was raised on a small ranch in rural Wyoming (which part of Wyoming isn't rural?), and spending $95,000 for six weeks of treatment at Menninger was not an option for him. However, he did have health insurance. Due to his diagnosis and other factors, Pasadena Villa in eastern Tennessee was the perfect fit. When it came to coming up with a $2,800 deposit for room and board, however, I simply said, "Not possible. If that's nonnegotiable, then James will have to go somewhere else."

Fortunately, Pasadena Villa stepped up to the plate and waived the room and board fee. James said he had never been to a place more beautiful, peaceful, and caring. I appreciate rehabs that are willing to make it work for a client. In addition to the quality of their treatment and commitment to integrity, it is one of the reasons I'll keep coming back to them.

I chalk up the following experience as "fool me once, shame on you, but fool me twice? That isn't gonna happen."

Three years ago, I sent a patient with alcohol addiction to a world-famous rehab. When I asked for the number of days his insurance company has been authorizing for residential treatment, I was told to expect no less than twenty-one days before they would step him down to PHP. After that, his room and board would be $200 per day for the remaining nine days of residential ($1,800). Not bad considering it could have been a lot worse.

Well, it was a lot worse. Imagine the shock I felt when the facility called me to say the insurance company was covering only six days of residential—six days including three days of detox! My client's counselor said that Magellan was only authorizing that number of days. "Magellan! What the hell does Magellan have to do with my client? His insurance is Blue Shield of California!" I exclaimed. This was when I discovered that Blue Shield of California contracts with Magellan to be the deliverer of bad news when it comes to cutting off authorized days of treatment. But why wasn't I told that? My discussions with the rehab were specifically regarding Blue Shield of California. Never once was Magellan brought up. If it had, my client would have gone to a different rehab!

As a result, we arrived at two understandings—a drastic reduction in the price of room and board and an increase of PHP days to make up for the loss of residential days. And I resolved to never use rehabs in business with Magellan.

Now you know why today receiving ninety days of treatment totally covered by your insurance at most rehabs is a pipedream. It's as if for years you faithfully pay your premiums, but when you need it, they dare you to use it. Ironically, the victim is victimized a second time—this time by the insurance company.

In- or Out-of-Network

Obviously, in today's world of health insurance, one really has to pay attention. But you are forgiven if you are confused and angered by the politics and how disrespectfully our lives are being treated. With what's going on in Washington, DC, who knows whether your current insurance will still be available next month? Welcome to the club. It's shameful.

Nonetheless, there are basically five ways rehabs deal with health insurance:

1. In-network means that a rehab and an insurance carrier have previously agreed on a schedule of reimbursement rates for all levels of treatment. The insurance company sends those reimbursements directly to the rehab.
2. Out-of-network means there is no set agreement; however, the insurance company and the rehab will negotiate reimbursement rates prior to treatment—usually settling on rates higher than in-network reimbursement rates. The deductible and out-of-pocket maximum are always higher (frequently two times higher) at an out-of-network facility—a tool the insurance company uses to steer beneficiaries to a facility where lower reimbursement rates have already been negotiated.

3. The rehab accepts private pay only, but as a courtesy, they will file out-of-network claims with your insurance company for you.
4. The rehab accepts private pay only, but they will direct you to a third party that for a fee will file your claims and try to get the maximum reimbursements for you.
5. The rehab accepts private pay only, and when it comes to insurance, you're on your own when it comes to filing claims.

It's a contradiction, but I frequently have made a better deal for my client with a rehab that is out-of-network with my client's insurance company than if they were in-network. The insurance company's reimbursement rates paid to a facility that is out-of-network are typically much higher than if they were in-network. In addition, the beneficiary's deductible and out-of-pocket maximum are always higher—frequently double. If I can get the facility to accept the lower in-network deductible and out of pocket, which has to be paid upfront by my client, it's a win-win for both parties since the higher out-of-network reimbursement fees more than make up the difference.

My client gets top-of-the-line treatment at a facility that normally is out of reach per his resources but is still using his insurance policy. The facility wins since they are getting higher than in-network reimbursement rates from an insurance carrier with whom they are out-of-network.

One reason I am able to make such favorable deals with the right rehabs is simple: rehabs see me as a steady source of clients who are the right fit, and I don't ask them for anything in return, other than giving my clients best treatment possible. They like the fact that I am not one of those scumbags who asks for a referral fee. They wouldn't do it anyway. They'd tell me to take a hike—and they'd be right to do so.

Unfortunately, making favorable deals for my clients with an out-of-network facility is getting progressively more difficult—if not impossible. Increasingly, if an individual has a non-employer-sponsored policy obtained through the Healthcare.gov exchange (the website where consumers can shop for and enroll in a health insurance program of their choice subsidized through the Affordable Care Act of 2010) or privately through a broker, in several states it is now common for the carrier to eliminate the cap on one's out-of-pocket spending when receiving treatment at an out-of-network facility. Generally, employer-sponsored policies maintain the cap on out-of-network out-of-pocket maximums.

What does that mean? It means that with that type of policy in certain states you are constrained to getting care at only facilities that are in-network with the insurance carrier. If you do get treatment at an out-of-network facility, the deductible is still higher, but now there is no maximum on your out-of-pocket amount—it is unlimited. You may as well be a private-pay patient. If your treatment is insurance dependent, the incentive to get care at an out-of-network facility is limited or not happening at all.

Insurance Dos and Don'ts

Helen Darling, the former head of the National Business Group on Health, summed up today's families' living situation this way:

> Soaring deductibles and medical bills are pushing millions of American families to the breaking point, fueling an affordability crisis that is pulling in middle-class households with health insurance as well as the poor and uninsured. Nearly half of those in a plan with at least $3,000 individual deductible or a $5,000 family deductible reported problems affording healthcare. In the real world, average people are living paycheck to paycheck. The whole situation drives me nuts.[12]

My clients who need to use their health insurance policy to access SUD and/or mental health treatment all ask the same question: "What will my policy cover?" Sometimes, they don't like the answer.

The following is a list of some details I have seen trip up clients when it comes to covering SUD and/or mental health treatment:

- If your priority is your monthly premium, the lower the premium, the higher the deductible, and the maximum out of pocket. But how practical is that? Are you able to handle a $7,500 deductible and a $15,000 or $20,000 out-of-pocket maximum in times of need?

- It's a good idea to know which specialty treatment facilities are in-network. Do the policy's behavioral health benefits cover in-patient residential care, or just outpatient care? What is the coverage for detox, PHP, IOP, and OP treatment? What are the average number of days authorized for each level of treatment?

- I've seen co-pay schedules go from 10/90 to 50/50 until they reach the out-of-pocket maximum. The lower the co-pay amount (for which the policy holder is responsible), the more expensive the premium—and vice versa.

- If the patient pays premiums on a monthly basis, the rehab asks for at least the next month's premium to be paid before admission; the next ninety days paid upfront is even better.

- With relapse a frequent occurrence, it's not unusual for some policies to allow not more than one round of residential treatment within a calendar year. They are usually more lenient when it comes to PHP, IOP, and OP, but with residential being the second-most expensive level of treatment, that's a different story. What will your policy allow?

- For those with a whole or sizeable unmet deductible and out-of-pocket maximum and entering rehab in November or December for a treatment regimen longer than thirty or sixty days, your deductible and out-of-pocket maximum will reset at the first of the next year and are subject to be paid upfront once again. I've witnessed people delaying admission to rehab until after the first of the year to avoid paying the deductible and out-of-pocket maximum twice within months of each other.

- Additionally, with co-payments increasing for ER visits, the insurance companies' intention is to steer those in need of immediate treatment to the less expensive emergency clinics.

Partial Hospitalization Programming (PHP)

Partial hospitalization programming (PHP) is residential treatment delivered on an outpatient basis. Frequently, it is referred to as "residential lite." Typically, PHP involves one or more of the following (see figure 5.12):

- Treatment continues as it has during the residential stage.
- Treatment continues at the same setting, but the patient is moved to off-campus housing, also called sober living.
- Treatment occurs at an off-campus clinic owned and operated by the facility or by an outside provider, and the patient moves to off-campus housing.

When PHP treatment occurs at an off-site, outpatient clinic, it is a milestone because the patient is leaving the cocoon of residential to now living in a separate sober living environment with others who are also transitioning back into "real life." The sober living house or apartment is typically off campus and owned and supervised by a third-party provider, although some rehabs will own and run their own.

While sober living is intended to be the first step in transitioning back into the "real world," the individual should remain in the sober living environment for a minimum of the remaining months of the one-year treatment plan. For those who are using medication-assisted therapy (MAT), finding a sober living house that allows it has been a challenge, but as MAT is becoming further

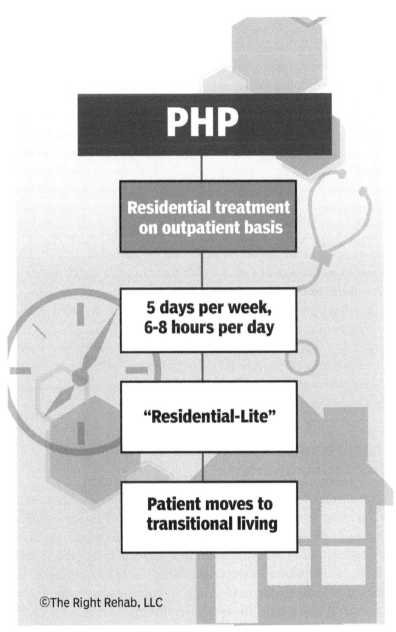

Figure 5.12.
Art © The Right Rehab, LLC.

blended into mainstream treatment, more sober living houses are accommodating its use.

The dilemma centers on the presence and use of any type of drug within the house that violates the fundamental sober living code of abstinence only. Furthermore, the once-banned medications are now an added responsibility of the house manager, who will have to secure medications on the premises—a formidable task in a house full of those with an addiction—plus control their dispensing.

Historically, PHP is the second thirty-day segment of a ninety-day treatment plan and is easily attainable at a private-pay facility. Usually, PHP comprises a total of fifteen to twenty sessions (five sessions per week over three or four five-day weeks) of six to eight hours each; the number of sessions could be extended if medically necessary and the patient's progress warrants it. On a cash basis, sessions can run from $250 to $850 each.

By using private pay, the facility is not tied to an insurance company's authorization for any level of treatment. The facility decides on a case-by-case basis the intensity of treatment a particular patient receives. The highly intensive RTC level of treatment could be longer than thirty days or shorter. Hence, the lower-intensity PHP could be started earlier or later than the thirty-day mark. See figure 5.13.

Partial Hospitalization Programming (PHP) When Using Insurance

As explained earlier in this chapter, if using insurance, plan on the insurance company stepping the patient down to PHP not at the beginning of the second thirty-day segment—day 31 of a ninety-day treatment plan—but instead anytime in what would normally be still in the residential phase of treatment. Since the insurance carrier is motivated to avoid paying residential's higher reimbursement rate at the soonest possible time, the facility in effect is stealing from PHP days to keep the patient under residential care at least through day 30. See figure 5.14.

Private pay allows 30 days RTC followed by 30 days outpatient PHP & sober living

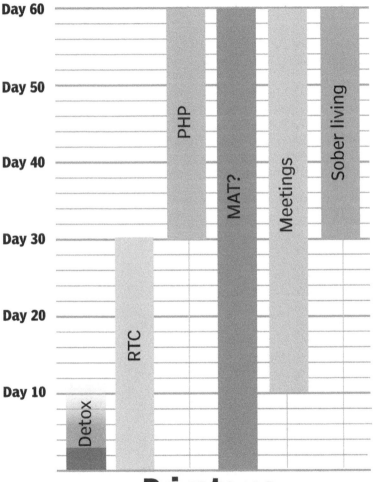

©The Right Rehab, LLC

Figure 5.13.

Art © The Right Rehab, LLC.

Insurance routinely stops RTC anytime after Day 10 to authorize less expensive PHP

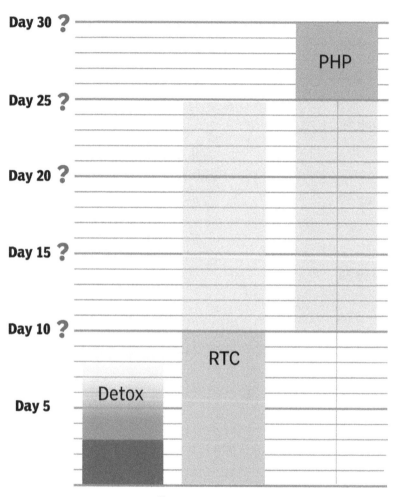

©The Right Rehab, LLC

Figure 5.14.

Art © The Right Rehab, LLC.

Typically, the patient doesn't notice that she has been stepped down to PHP from residential since she sleeps in the same bed and all continues the same since the first day of residential. The insurance company is still paying for treatment (albeit now at a lower rate to the facility), but more often than not, the facility begins charging for R&B (room and board). Not all rehabs pass along that charge, but since the insurance is supposed to reimburse only for the therapeutic portion of treatment after the residential stage, most facilities do charge since they are now receiving a lower reimbursement from the insurance carrier while still providing the same level of services. Depending on the facility, R&B rates can range from $25 to $300 per day.

As previously mentioned, in some states it is against state law to have PHP treatment and housing occur in the same setting, therefore, PHP patients must move to off-campus living. Again, it is my job to predict when that will happen with a particular rehab, so my client's financial guarantor is not surprised by a new charge.

Intensive Outpatient Programming (IOP)

Intensive Outpatient Programming (IOP) is a less intensive schedule of therapy that allows the individual to integrate further into the "real world." Continuing to reside in sober living, the individual has a choice of morning or evening sessions at a clinic or occasionally on-site to make time for getting a job, continuing education, or performing community service. At this stage of the treatment plan, the individual's social network of those living in sobriety is growing. New relationships and support are now becoming integral parts of the patient's life. See figure 5.15.

In keeping within a ninety-day private-pay schedule, sessions are two or three hours each, sometimes starting at five times, then four times, but mostly three times per week within a thirty-day window. The last session of IOP usually marks the end of formal treatment; however, for the remaining nine months of the one-year treatment

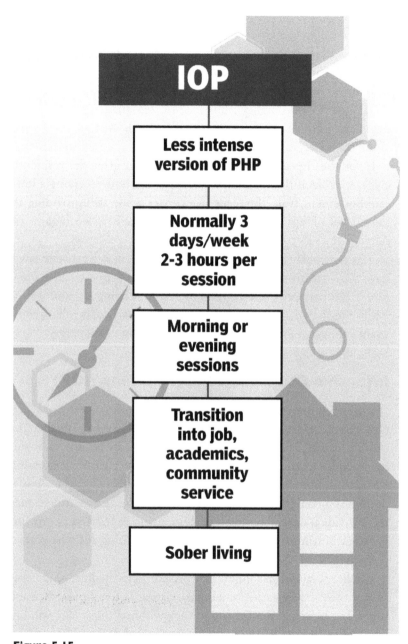

Figure 5.15.
Art © The Right Rehab, LLC.

plan, the individual continues employing a much wider form of recovery support services (RSS), including outpatient programming (OP) for one- or two-hour sessions once per week. Again, with a private-pay facility, the timing and number of sessions is at the total discretion of the facility and the patient. See figure 5.16.

The cash price of IOP can run from $50 to $400 per session depending on variables such as the particular programming and location. For insurance-driven patients, some rehabs will access a patient's IOP days in order to stretch the formal treatment period as long as possible. That means the insurance company stepping the patient down to IOP not at the beginning of the third thirty-day segment—day 61 of a ninety-day treatment plan—but earlier depending on how long the facility can stretch authorization for the previous PHP treatment. See figure 5.17.

The number of IOP sessions insurance allows is not set in stone. Like so many variables regarding insurance coverage, it depends on the state where the facility is located, the state where the policy is registered, and the relationship between the facility and the insurance company. I have experienced rehabs providing IOP between twelve and twenty-four sessions (three or four of them per a five-day week) over a four- to eight-week period. Again, the number of days to expect coverage could be less or more per the relationship between the insurance company and the facility.

The Takeaway Regarding Private Pay versus Insurance

Treatment at a specialty facility that includes RTC usually charges on a per-month basis. The total fee can be paid upfront—for which there is normally a slight discount—or one could set a payment schedule. I have worked with rehabs that charge anywhere from $5,000 to $80,000 per month. Nationwide, however, it is prudent to expect paying an average of $12,000 to $30,000 per month for a private-pay, thirty-day, sixty-day or ninety-day treatment protocol.

Patient continues residing in sober living during IOP, a less intensive schedule of treatment that fosters patient's transitioning into a fully functional and active life.

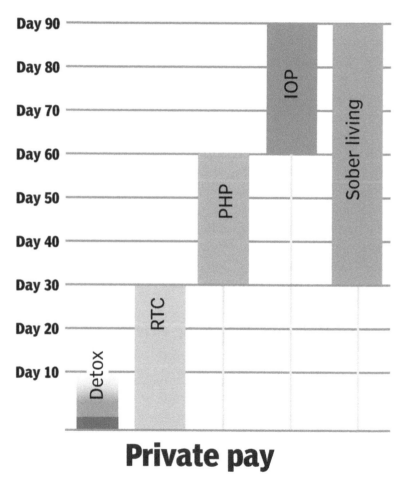

Figure 5.16.
Art © The Right Rehab, LLC.

With insurance-driven patients, some rehabs stretch PHP as long as possible and then start IOP to keep formal treatment going.

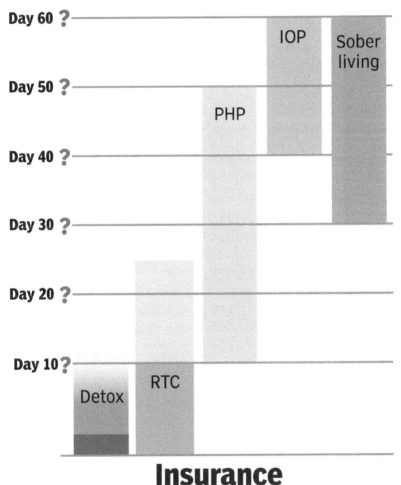

Figure 5.17.
Art © The Right Rehab, LLC.

As previously stated, treatment at a specialty facility, including RTC that is insurance driven, is totally dependent on the insurance company wanting to spend as little as possible on the more expensive stages for which the insurance company has to reimburse the facility—detox, RTC, PHP, and IOP. The number of treatment days are inconsistent from facility to facility depending on the location of the rehab, the state where the policy is written, the policy itself, and the relationship between the rehab and the insurance carrier. Basically, the days covered are all over the map, but they are almost always under the ninety days that you get with private pay.

Recovery Support Services (RSS)

After ninety days of formal treatment, RSS is the continuing care or aftercare balance of a one-year (and hopefully lifetime-long) treatment plan. "These supportive services are typically delivered by trained case managers, recovery coaches, and/or peers. RSS can be effective in promoting healthy lifestyle techniques to increase resilience skills, reduce the risk of relapse and help those affected by substance use disorders achieve and maintain recovery."[13] See figure 5.18.

Recovery support is exactly that—a foundation in maintaining sobriety, preventing relapse, and living a lifestyle of recovery for a lifetime. There are several sources supporting for that, including the following:

- Outpatient programming (OP) that steps down group to one hour per week of organized group therapy
- Private sessions with a psychologist or licensed counselor if possible
- Continued living in a sober living environment
- Peer support, including continuous attendance at twelve-step or other type of support group
- Job search or job training
- Continued education

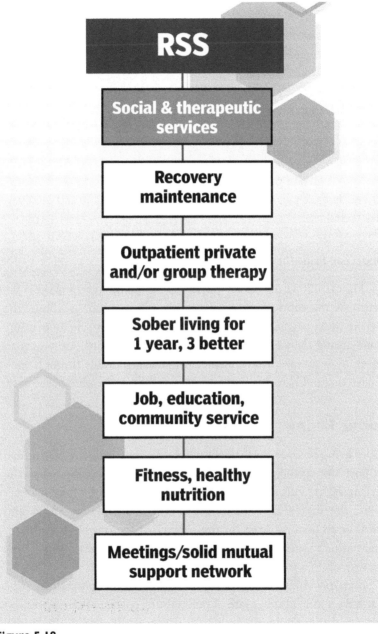

Figure 5.18.
Art © The Right Rehab, LLC.

- Healthy nutrition
- Transportation availability
- Legal assistance
- Community service
- Fitness
- Childcare, if necessary for employment

One-Year Plan—Private Pay

When private pay is the source of treatment, figure 5.19 depicts how adherence to a one-year treatment plan is possible and relatively easy to follow.

One-Year Plan—Insurance

Figure 5.20 visualizes how insurance-dependent treatment is the victim of the capriciousness of the insurance company. Thus, the patient must be nimble and ready for a change in schedule at any point during the treatment period. A straightforward one-year plan driven by insurance can be challenging but achievable through one's persistence and hard work to maintain and thrive in a life of sobriety.

Sober Living

Sober living provides both a substance-free environment and mutual support among fellow residents (see figure 5.21). Ideally, when the patient starts with the outpatient treatment stage of formal treatment, the individual should reside at a sober living setting and continue to do so at least for the balance of the one-year treatment plan—nine months after formal treatment—and then optimally all the way up to a total of three years.

Statistics show that those who stay in sober living for at least one year have a much higher rate of maintaining sobriety than those who don't, and the rate is still higher if the stay is three years. Additionally, one trial found that those with severe SUDs who lived in sober

Private pay offers the most freedom when executing a one-year plan of conventional treatment and recovery support services (RSS).

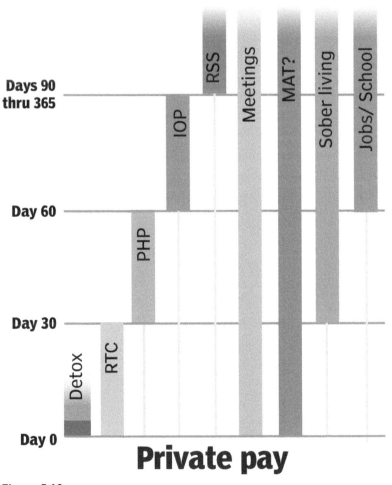

Figure 5.19.
Art © The Right Rehab, LLC.

Insurance-dependent treatment is constantly adjusting within the confines of insurance authorization. 90 days covered by insurance is now virtually impossible.

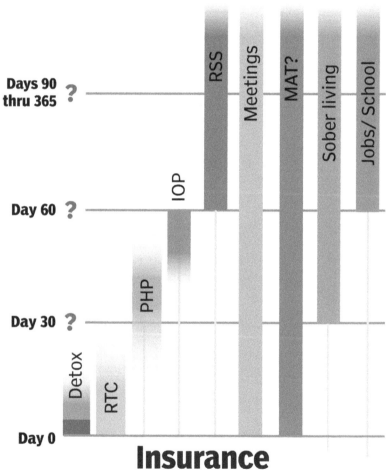

Figure 5.20.

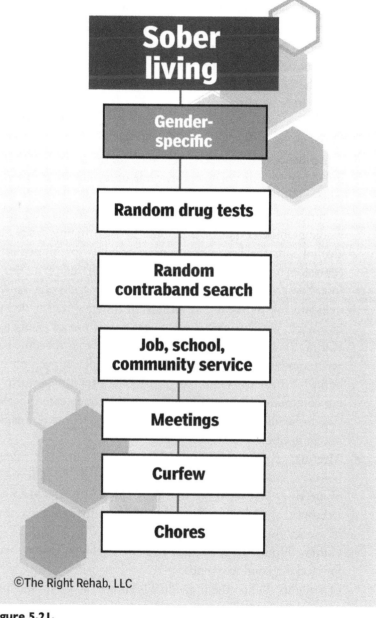

©The Right Rehab, LLC

Figure 5.21.
Art © The Right Rehab, LLC.

living after treatment "were 2 times more likely to be abstinent and had higher monthly incomes and lower incarceration rates"[14] two years later versus those who did not reside in sober living.

No matter where a sober living residence may be located throughout the country, there are several principles that the ones with integrity have in common:

- Drug testing: Random drug tests are universal, although consequences for a positive test vary. Some houses expel an individual for one positive test, while others institute a more lenient and progressive policy.
- Contraband search: Searches of individual rooms and the whole premises occur on a random basis. Bringing drugs or alcohol into the house is normally grounds for immediate expulsion, although different places have different penalties.
- Job: Every house with which I am familiar has the same mandate for those not in all-day treatment—if you don't have a job, you have two weeks to get one. If you are going to IOP, OP, or individual counseling, arrange your schedule to accommodate all activities. If you're not employed, you must be in job training, continuing your education, or performing community service. Lounging on the couch eating See's Candies while watching *Married . . . with Children* reruns is not an option.
- Meetings: Again, different residences have different rules; however, most houses mandate attendance at a set number of meetings per week, whether these are AA, NA, SMART Recovery, or Celebrate Recovery. If the individual does not have a sponsor, it's time to get one.
- Curfew: Hours the individual must be in the residence vary for weekdays and weekends.
- Overnights: When the individual is allowed to spend one or more nights outside of the residence, it's usually a privilege

earned, as well as a result of how much time the person has been a resident and obedient of the house rules.

Medication-Assisted Therapy (MAT)

"Medication-assisted treatment saves lives while increasing the chances a person will remain in treatment and learn the skills and build the networks necessary for long-term recovery."

—Michael Botticelli, director of National Drug Control Policy[15]

Controversial in some circles, a lifesaver in others, MAT is a "combination of behavioral interventions and medications to treat substance use disorders that studies have repeatedly demonstrated its efficacy at reducing illicit drug use and overdose deaths."[16] These are not magic pills that "cure" addiction, but medications combined with evidence-based therapies have proven to produce higher rates of remission, shrink the gap between treatment need and availability, incur lower costs of treatment than without it, and reduce the rates of relapse, cravings, and risk of death due to overdose.

MAT alone is not treatment or a substitute for it. However, because some of the medications are opioids themselves, MAT is directly contrary to the abstinence-only ethos and, therefore, has its considerable critics. Out of 15,961 treatment programs surveyed by the Substance Abuse and Mental Health Services Administration (SAMHSA), just 7,770 (48.7 percent) utilize any form of MAT.[17]

Once a person becomes addicted, the driving force behind the continued use of a substance is to get through or even out the peaks and valleys of the effects in order to avoid withdrawal. Medications approved by the Food and Drug Administration (FDA) are used to smooth out those highs and lows so that the victim can effectively get through the day without resorting to illicit substances and all the destructive elements that come along with it. As a substitute for illicit opioids, MAT's introduction into the treatment regimen inherently contributes to a reduction in the transmission of HIV, hepatitis C, and other infectious diseases; overall criminal activity and the associated criminal justice and social costs; and, of course, overdose deaths.

It is argued that taking meds for SUD is similar to taking medication for any other disease. "In some ways, MAT is like insulin for patients with diabetes. Whether treating diabetes or substance use disorder, medications are best employed as part of a broader treatment plan involving behavioral health therapies and RSS, as well as regular monitoring."[18] See figure 5.22.

Like SUD treatment, there is no "one-size-fits-all" approach with MAT. People benefit from it for varying lengths of time; therefore, its use must be based on the individual's needs. The best results occur when a patient receives medication for as long as it provides a benefit, which is called "maintenance treatment."[19]

To be effective, maintenance treatment should not be fewer than ninety days, and one study suggests that individuals who receive MAT for fewer than three years are more likely to relapse than those who benefit from its treatment for three or more years.[20] Ultimately, the individual could continue using MAT and slowly taper off at a time of his choosing or continue its use for the rest of his lifetime.

The three medications commonly used for opioid addiction are the following (see figure 5.23):

- *Methadone* is a synthetic opioid that has been used for more than forty years to treat withdrawal symptoms chiefly from heroin use. Methadone is an agonist, meaning it activates one's opioid receptors but blocks an opioid's euphoric effect and reduces withdrawal and cravings. Studies show that methadone produces a treatment retention rate higher than treatment without medication. Patients on methadone were four times more likely to stay in treatment and have 33 percent fewer opioid-positive drug tests compared to those treated with a placebo.[21]

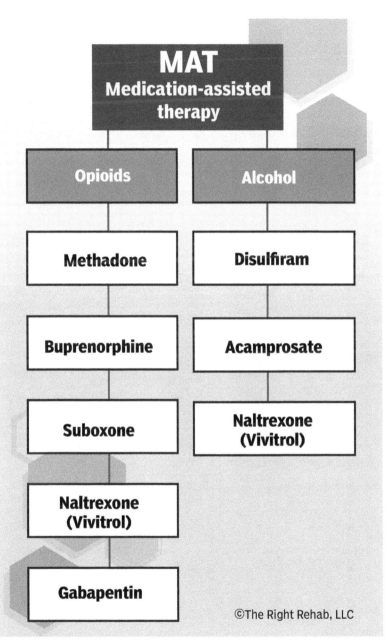

Figure 5.22.
Art ©The Right Rehab, LLC.

FDA Approved Drugs for MAT

Medication	Action	Method	Dosing	Location
Methadone	**Full Agonist:** Generates Effect	Pill, Liquid	Daily	Opioid Treatment Program
Buprenorphine	**Partial Agonist:** Limited Effect	Pill or Film*	Daily	Any prescriber with Appropriate Waiver
		Under-skin Implant	Every 6 Months	
Naltrexone	**Antagonist:** Blocks Effect	Oral	Daily	Any prescriber with Authority
		Extended-Release Injectable	Monthly	

* Placed inside the cheek or under the tongue.

Source: 2016 The Pew Charitable Trust

©The Right Rehab, LLC

Figure 5.23.
Source: Pew Charitable Trusts (2016). Art © The Right Rehab, LLC.

Downsides of methadone include its need to be administered every twenty-four to thirty-six hours at a federally approved clinic, the chance of misuse and overdose, and likely accompanying constipation, vomiting, sweating, dizziness, and sedation.

- *Buprenorphine* is a partial agonist, meaning it activates opioid receptors—not enough to produce a "high," but enough to reduce withdrawal and craving. In order to start a treatment regimen, the individual must be in withdrawal with the previous illicit opioid's effect subsided.

  Buprenorphine has a ceiling effect, meaning that its effects will plateau and will not increase even with repeated dosing. It won't produce euphoria and does not have some of the dangerous side effects associated with other opioids. Multiple studies found that patients using buprenorphine showed a 75–80 percent reduction in positive opioid test results.

  One downside is withdrawal that comes after abrupt termination of its use. Other side effects include constipation, vomiting, headache, sweating, insomnia, and blurred vision. Once the decision is made to discontinue its treatment, the process of safely tapering the dose often spans many months.[22]

- *Naltrexone* (Vivitrol) is an "antagonist" since it blocks the opioid receptors to block their activation and, thus, prohibits the euphoric effects of opioids. It also interrupts the effects of any opioids in a person's system, precipitating an opioid withdrawal syndrome in opioid-dependent patients, so it can be administered only after a complete detoxification from opioids.[23]

  Since any euphoric effect is prevented by naltrexone, there is no physical dependence associated with its use. Therefore, it is recommended for relapse prevention and abstinence-based treatment, not for withdrawal management like methadone and buprenorphine.

The following medications used to treat alcohol addiction do not present a risk of misuse or addiction:

- *Disulfiram* acts as a deterrent to drinking alcohol since it causes severe physical reactions when mixed with alcohol. Effects range from nausea, vomiting, sweating, dizziness, heart palpitations, and headache.
- *Acamprosate* does not produce a reaction to alcohol intake but reduces symptoms of craving in order to prevent relapse. Research shows that it works best with those who maintain a motivation to remain abstinent when used with ongoing counseling.
- *Naltrexone* (Vivitrol) is the same opioid antagonist used to treat opioid use disorder (OUD) that blocks opioid receptors. It does not cause severe reactions to alcohol intake, but it still prohibits its euphoric or pleasurable effects.

Scientific evidence suggests that relapse rates are high when tapering off these medications and treatment programs too early. It is often the case that patients with good long-term outcomes are the ones who engaged in MAT, although cycling in and out of treatment is not unusual in the path to stable recovery. Maintenance treatments have also been shown to reduce injection drug use and HIV transmission and to be protective against overdose.[24]

Despite the encouraging statistics of remission and its cost-effectiveness, currently roughly half of specialty treatment programs do not integrate MAT into their treatment regimens. There persists a hesitation to implement MAT due to the belief that since they are opioids, it simply means replacing one set of opioids with another. True. MAT utilizes opioids, but ones that prevent the use and downstream effects (and potential deaths due to overdose) of illicit opioids like heroin and fentanyl. Some maintain that increased medication access is key in successful treatment.

The cycle of euphoria, crash, and craving—sometimes repeated several times a day—is a hallmark of addiction and results in severe behavioral disruption. These characteristics result from heroin's rapid onset and short duration of action in the brain. In contrast, methadone and buprenorphine have gradual onsets of action and produce stable levels of the drug in the brain. As a result, patients maintained on these medications do not experience a rush, while they also markedly reduce their desire to use opioids.[25]

German Lopez wrote in one of his pieces for *Vox*, "Behind the arguments about MAT is a simple reality of how Americans view addiction: many still don't see it, as public health experts do, as a disease."[26] Lopez so perfectly illustrated that ignorance by reprinting a letter he received from a reader:

> Darwin's Theory says, "survival of the fittest." Let those lost souls pay the price of their criminal choices and criminal actions. Society does not owe them multiple medical resuscitations from their own bad judgment, criminal activity and self-inflicted wounds.[27]

> "Such views are not scientifically supported since the research clearly demonstrates that MAT leads to better treatment outcomes compared to behavioral treatments alone. . . . In fact, ample research shows that, when used correctly, MAT can reduce or eliminate illicit drug use, associated criminality, infectious disease transmission and restore patients to healthy functioning."

> —Vivek H. Murthy (MD, MBA),
> U.S. surgeon general, 2014–2017, 2021–[28]

Mutual-Aid Support Groups

> I was always the black sheep. Then I started going to meetings and found the rest of the herd.[29]

Alcoholics Anonymous (AA) is the precursor of today's recovery support services (RSS). Founded in 1935 by Bill Wilson and Bob

Smith in Akron, Ohio, the group states that its purpose is to enable "its members to stay sober and help other alcoholics achieve sobriety."[30] Since mainstream medical and psychiatric practice did not treat alcohol addiction as a chronic disease at that time—if treated at all, it was in asylums and not a part of mainstream health care—AA members took it upon themselves to help treat each other. It wasn't until 1956 that the American Medical Association (AMA) declared alcoholism an illness.

Not to be mistaken as a substitute for treatment, twelve-step self-help groups such as AA are integral to a person's aftercare in maintaining sobriety and living a life in recovery. Its mutual support is based on members sharing a problem, and through experiential knowledge and peer support, they learn from each other and focus on personal-change goals. AA is built on two guiding principles—a twelve-step plan of action and the existence of a higher power than oneself—and studies show that 50 percent of those who started attending AA meetings after formal treatment are still participating in meetings three years later.[31]

Benefits of participation in AA and NA include lower health care costs associated with relapses; help for members to cope with awkward social situations, depression, and cravings; and support from other members in getting through exceedingly difficult times when one's reaction was once use of substances. Most of those whom I know in recovery insist that a lifetime adherence to AA's twelve-step program and meetings is essential for their ongoing recovery.

Although AA is the most well known of mutual support or self-help programs, it certainly is not the only one; others include Narcotics Anonymous (NA), Al-Anon, Cocaine Anonymous (CA), SMART Recovery, and Celebrate Recovery.

Three key ideas predominate in effective twelve-step programs:

- *Acceptance* includes the realization that drug addiction is a chronic, progressive disease over which one has no control, that life has become unmanageable because of drugs or alcohol, that willpower alone is insufficient to overcome the problem, and that abstinence is the only alternative.

- *Surrender* involves giving oneself over to a higher power, accepting the fellowship and support structure of other recovering addicted individuals, and following the recovery activities laid out by the twelve-step program.
- *Active involvement* in twelve-step meetings and related activities. While the efficacy of twelve-step programs in treating alcohol dependence has been established, the research on its usefulness for other forms of substance abuse is more preliminary, but the treatment appears promising for helping drug users sustain recovery.[32]

The Family Must Also Be in Recovery

"Structured Family Recovery transforms recovery into a shared journey the family takes together with the newly recovering alcoholic or addict."

—Debra Jay[33]

I see this all the time: A family member goes away to treatment—whether it be thirty, sixty, or ninety days or longer—and when he returns, the family expects him to be "fixed." Presto, no more addiction, and no more problems. Trust me, it doesn't work like that. So often, treatment professionals and I have met patients' family members and thought, "Oh, now I see the problem."

The point is that, in so many cases, a person's addiction/mental disorder is a manifestation of what's going on at home. So, it's not just the patient who needs to do the work; the family unit has to work on itself as well. What good does it do for the patient to do all the work while the other half of the equation does nothing?

This is why when I send someone to treatment who is part of a family unit, I set up that family to see a specialist who will be in communication with the patient's therapist at the facility. That's in addition to family therapy sessions that occur usually once per week with the patient and his therapist. Only when the family unit owns its role in the recovery process will the individual and the family be on a path to recovery. You can't have one without the other.

If you are part of a family that has a member in treatment or recovery, do yourself a favor and read the book that is universally acclaimed as the best one on this subject: *It Takes a Family* by Debra Jay. She not only explains why the family's role is key but also shows the family the work that must be done and how to do it.

There are also self-help groups that help family members understand the family member's disease. Al-Anon is a mutual-aid group that does exactly that; the group fosters emotional stability for the family member and encourages "loving detachment" from the loved one rather than coaching members to "get their loved one into treatment and recovery." Clinical trials and other studies show that participating family members experience reduced depression, anger, and relationship unhappiness at rates and levels comparable to those receiving psychological therapy.[34] It's useful to mention that 80 percent of Al-Anon's members happen to be female.

Relapse

> More than 60% of people treated for SUD relapse within the first year of discharge from treatment and remain at increased risk of relapse for many years.[35]

Often relapse occurs when the person is doing well with recovery. The individual may remember the halcyon days of her substance use, even though it may have been a long time ago, when her use didn't cause problems. Frequently, the person wishes to return to that place, but this is impossible since addiction changes the physical makeup of the brain. Today, the person in recovery is no longer the same person who was able to use drugs or alcohol in a controlled fashion. See figure 5.24.

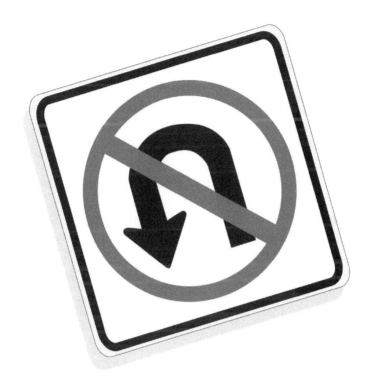

RELAPSE

The **return** to drug use after a significant period of **abstinence.**

Figure 5.24.
Art © The Right Rehab, LLC.

Professional caregivers with decades of experience working with those affected by SUD—and in decades of long-term recovery themselves—say that when one relapses, it is crucial to determine what's changed and what could have triggered the break from sobriety. Concurrently, the relapsed victim must start immediately with one or more of the following:

- The individual's total dedication to sobriety and eventual recovery is priority one.
- The person must reinstate treatment per the severity of the relapse, but with adjustments based on what is known at that point.
- The individual should consider instituting medication-assisted therapy (MAT) if it's not already being used.
- The individual must be living in an environment conducive to a lifestyle of recovery.

It's not an anomaly for victims to go through multiple treatment programs before they finally "get it." Karin Swenson, a prominent treatment executive, puts it this way when it comes to relapse: "It's one thing to know the tools, but sometimes you need help remembering how to use them."[36]

For most families, however, multiple rehab stays are not even a choice since the first round of treatment usually consumes all available resources—with or without insurance. A common refrain I hear when families are sending a loved one to treatment is "Better make this one work, because the next one is on you."

HOW TO GET TREATMENT

"The true measure of any society can be found in how it treats its most vulnerable members."

—Mohandas Gandhi[1]

What? They Want *How Much* for Treatment?

In 2019, 61.2 million of us eighteen or older had either substance use disorder (SUD) or mental illness—9.5 million had both (see figure 6.1). Of the 20.4 million people who needed SUD treatment, only 4.2 million actually received it; 2.6 million (4 percent of us) received treatment at a specialty facility (a hospital, rehab or mental health center). Slightly more than 20 percent of our fellow citizens had a mental illness—that's 51.7 million—yet more than half (thirty-four million) did *not* get treatment.[2]

Why didn't those who needed (or at least wanted) treatment actually get it? Very few can afford to pay $15,000 to $80,000 per month out of their own pocket for treatment at a rehab facility. For most of us, even if it's remotely possible, it's impossible to justify those costs—if it's not the price of a home, it is at least the down payment.

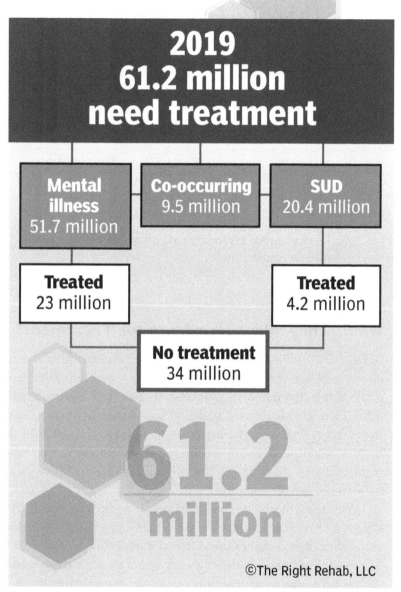

Figure 6.1.

Source: Substance Abuse and Mental Health Services Administration, "Key Substance Use and Mental Health Indicators in the United States" (2020). Art © The Right Rehab, LLC.

However, if at all possible, one way to justify coming up with such a large sum—it's all relative—is to ask whether the patient were to live a normal life span (into one's eighties or nineties). Now, amortize the cost of treatment over the years to get there. It puts a different spin on the cost factor. It's not so many dollars per year in exchange for living a hopefully full, productive life over the next forty or fifty years—if one is a millennial. Those who are able will do it for a house, a car, or a college education. What's a life worth?

Plus, if you figure the expense of substance abuse to the individual—the cost of the substance, the health care costs that are three times higher, likely criminal justice costs, possible incarceration, family/social/career losses, and possible early death—the high cost of treatment may not be such a bad deal.

In fact, according to a study done by researchers at the University of Illinois, Chicago, it's damn expensive to be a heroin addict. The annual societal cost of the more than one million heroin users in the United States was $51.2 billion (in 2015 dollars). Of that $51.2 billion, 42.3 percent—or about $20,000 of the $50,799 cost per person—is just the direct cost to the user for heroin purchases. The downstream costs—productivity loss, drug treatment, health care–related costs, and crime—make up the rest.[3]

So often I've seen parents and grandparents go through a child's college fund, take out an equity loan on their house, or pillage retirement funds—all to send a child to treatment. It makes you ill to see this happen, and then to see the child relapse, as the majority of them do, becomes too much to take.

For those who live paycheck to paycheck, unless there's a Robin Hood in one's life, private pay for ninety days of formal treatment at a rehab is likely not going to happen.

One thing to be clear about, however, is that although resources play a crucial role, they alone don't get the victim sober. Ultimately, it's the individual who decides that. A beachfront estate, celebrity chef meals, equine therapy, daily massages, a sweat lodge, acupuncture, private projection room, and a sober companion are not necessary tools for getting sober. I have worked with drug users and drunks who finally "get it"—from trust-fund babies and self-made, outrageously financially successful people who go through multiple rehabs of the most expensive kind to those who don't have two nickels to rub together.

Some of the most successful outcomes are those whose treatment is paid for by an employer, state government, county court (for court-ordered treatment), or public assistance (e.g., charities, private scholarship funds, etc.) or is free at AA meetings. Why does one particular treatment eventually work for an individual? I think it's that the victim eventually realizes that there are only two options—sobriety or death. Only then can one take full advantage of the treatment available to lead one down the right path.

So, what options are left if one doesn't have access to private-pay resources, employer-based coverage, or a private health insurance policy? Since that road to recovery is out of reach for most who need it, one must find the road that matches one's resources.

Fortunately, there are routes, but it takes work—and, most of all, commitment—to carve one's own path through the Khyber Pass of addiction and onward into the promised land of recovery. Like water seeking its own level, one can find the means that work. A good place to start is determining one's resources and knowing the programs that fit those resources.

Just as there are several different substance-related maladies, there are several facilities where one may go to treat them (see figure 6.2). Outpatient treatment wins the day when it comes to the type of care most prevalent—more than 66 percent of specialty programs offer outpatient treatment in the form of detox, partial hospitalization programing (PHP), intensive outpatient programing (IOP), regular outpatient programming (OP), and medication-assisted therapy (MAT). They are also ultimately the most affordable and accessible.

More than likely, there is an outpatient program that fits one's resources. One person could be starting out only with donations of $10 or $50; one might be able to afford to pay insurance co-pays; and perhaps another can pay fees of $500 per session privately.

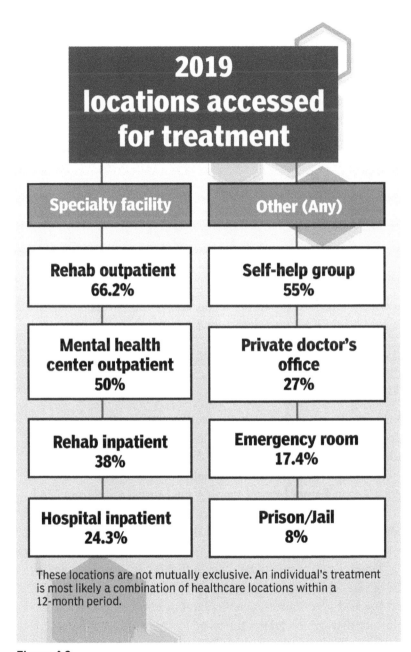

2019 locations accessed for treatment

Specialty facility	Other (Any)
Rehab outpatient 66.2%	Self-help group 55%
Mental health center outpatient 50%	Private doctor's office 27%
Rehab inpatient 38%	Emergency room 17.4%
Hospital inpatient 24.3%	Prison/Jail 8%

These locations are not mutually exclusive. An individual's treatment is most likely a combination of healthcare locations within a 12-month period.

Figure 6.2.

Source: Substance Abuse and Mental Health Services Administration, "Locations Received Illicit Drug Use Treatment in Past Year among Persons Aged 12 or Older Who Received Illicit Drug Use Treatment at a Specialty Facility in Past Year by Percentages" (2020). Art © The Right Rehab, LLC.

Besides price, the key is finding the program that's the best fit for an individual situation, which depends on a number of variables:

- Location
- Schedule
- Treatment for a particular diagnosis
- Age, gender, and ethnicity
- Suicide attempts
- Ability to get social services such as medication, legal and financial counsel, employment, education, and childcare

When it comes to residential treatment, only 26 percent of programs offer non-hospital inpatient detox and residential programs. There are options for people with special needs that take into account an individual's medical condition or social/economic situation, options for active or retired service members, and options for age- and/or gender appropriate therapy.

Medicaid and Medicare

Do you know what resources are available and how to access them? Medicaid and Medicare could be two options depending on the individual situation.

Although I was just a kid, I'm old enough to remember President Lyndon Baines Johnson signing the legislation creating Medicare and Medicaid in 1965. Although at the time I didn't understand their purpose, millions of others did since that was the starting point of the federal government providing low-cost health care primarily for America's elderly population. Until then, if you were over the age of sixty-five (not old nor elderly by today's standards) and ill, and you had no resources, you were out of luck. Thanks to Lyndon Johnson, that was no longer the case.

"The 1962 publication of Michael Harrington's *The Other America*, an expose which demonstrated that poverty in America was far more prevalent than commonly assumed, focused public debate on the issue."[4] Fortunately, it inspired one reader to do something about it—President John F. Kennedy. "Harrington's book spurred Kennedy, and then Johnson, to formulate an anti-poverty agenda, on which Harrington consulted alongside Daniel Patrick Moynihan and Director of the Peace Corps, Sargent Shriver."[5]

In Sargent Shriver, Johnson entrusted his mothership of antipoverty programs—the Office of Economic Opportunity (OEO)—to lead the fight for Johnson's "Great Society." Within only sixty days (lightspeed then; impossible now), Shriver created life-changing programs for our fellow citizens desperately in need of a hand up—Head Start, Vista, Job Corps, Legal Services, Foster Grandparents, Upward Bound, and Neighborhood Health Services, to name just a few.

One result is "[t]hat government action is literally the only reason we have less poverty in 2012 than we did in 1967."[6] If there is anyone without "Saint" in front of their name who worked harder to improve the human condition more than Sargent Shriver, I'm not aware of them.

Medicare and Medicaid were created to be government-funded and government-supervised programs that serve two groups of Americans needing assistance in getting crucial health care that otherwise would not be available. Regardless of one's income, Medicare is a federal program providing health coverage for Americans sixty-five and older, as well as for those under sixty-five and disabled. Medicaid is a federal/state partnership providing health care coverage for low-income families.

Medicaid

Medicaid provides the primary health insurance coverage for low-income Americans between the ages of nineteen and sixty-four years old. As of May 2020, Medicaid and the Children's Health Insurance Program (CHIP) covered more than 73,469,597 low-income children, pregnant women, adults, seniors, and people with disabilities.

Covering in excess of 20 percent (or one in five) of Americans, it's also responsible for 20 percent of all health care spending in the United States, including major funding for hospitals, community health centers, and nursing homes.

Funded through a partnership between the federal government and individual states, the federal government matches each dollar spent by a state, plus any additional amount per a set formula to cover a particular state's costs for citizens requiring health care. Though each state designs its own program, the federal government's share of funding for states has been anywhere from at least 50 percent to 77 percent for poorer states.

Who Qualifies for Medicaid?

So, you may now be thinking, "Okay, Medicaid sounds like it could be the answer to getting SUD treatment for myself or a loved one, but how does one get it?"

If you have not been living under a rock, lately you may have heard the terms *SSI*, *FPL*, *ACA*, and *Medicaid expansion*. If you or a family member needs substance use disorder treatment or just general health care, the following is important to know.

Supplemental Security Income (SSI)

In most states, individuals who have a mental illness could be eligible for supplemental security income (SSI), the federal cash assistance program for low-income aged, blind, or disabled individuals. By being in that program, an individual is also automatically eligible for Medicaid. To be eligible for SSI, individuals must have low incomes, limited assets, and an impaired ability to work at a substantial gainful level as a result of old age or significant disability. However, SUD is not considered a disability for purposes of qualifying for SSI.[7]

You could contact an insurance broker or the Social Security Administration to see which, if any, Social Security programs you or a loved one qualify for: 1-800-772-1213 or https://www.ssa.gov/.

Federal Poverty Level (FPL)

FPL is "a measure of [household] income" issued every year by the Department of Health and Human Services (HHS) that is used to determine your eligibility for certain programs and benefits, including the following:

- the Marketplace insurance (the Affordable Care Act or Obamacare)
- Medicaid and CHIP (Children's Health Insurance Program)

Household income is defined as the total income of "yourself, your spouse if you're married, plus everyone you'll claim as a tax dependent, including those who don't need coverage."[8] In practical terms, the FPL is the baseline, the minimum amount of income necessary for sole persons and families to cover room and board, clothes, and transportation in our country—Alaska and Hawaii have higher rates due to their higher costs of living.

How Do I Determine My Income?

To know whether you qualify for Medicaid (or any other government program, for that matter), you start with last year's 1040 Federal Tax form, which you reported (hopefully) to the Internal Revenue Service (IRS). On line 7 is your adjusted gross income (AGI). Based on that year's AGI, estimate your expected AGI for the year you want insurance coverage to begin—that is usually the end of the current year. Starting with your estimated AGI, we estimate your MAGI.

Your MAGI is the total of the following for each member of your household who's required to file a tax return:

- Your adjusted gross income (AGI) on your federal tax return
- Excluded foreign income
- Nontaxable Social Security benefits (including tier 1 railroad retirement benefits)

- Tax-exempt interest
- MAGI does not include Supplemental Security Income (SSI)[9]

The term *MAGI* is not on your 1040 Federal Tax form, but, as stated previously, it's very similar to your adjusted gross income (AGI), which is on line 7 of your 1040 Federal Tax form.

Don't worry—you're not going to prison if the expected income you estimate is not the same as the actual figure you report on your next tax return. You will be assessed later with a larger allowance if you underestimated your expected MAGI, or else you will owe the difference on your next tax return if you overestimated it. No biggie. Since I don't even pretend to be a tax expert, you'd be smart to ask an accountant and/or visit these two websites: https://www.healthcare .gov/income-and-household-information/how-to-report/ and https:// www.healthcare.gov/income-and-household-information/how-to -report/#dontknowAGI. Since it will be difficult to determine your income if you are unemployed, visit https://www.healthcare.gov/ unemployed/coverage/#unemployedincome. If you are self-employed, visit https://www.healthcare.gov/self-employed/income/.

The Affordable Care Act (ACA) and Medicaid Expansion

Here's the problem: substance addiction costs our country at least $700 billion to $1 trillion a year in health care, law enforcement, and criminal justice, and that's not including the tragic consequences for our family and social structures. Inexplicably, substance use disorder treatment is out of reach for way too many of us due to the lack of health insurance coverage.

One proven answer: make health insurance available and afford-able to those who need it because a healthy citizen is a productive citizen—and, ultimately, a tax-paying citizen.

Despite the passage of Medicaid in 1966, there still were too many Americans not receiving coverage, which, in 2013, translated to more than 48.6 million people, or 18 percent of the U.S. population. Medicaid was available to children, low-income adults with dependent children, pregnant women, adults with disabilities, and certain people over sixty-five. Medicaid, however, did not cover adults *without* dependent children. That's a problem since "among uninsured adults (especially young adult males), 12% met DSM-IV criteria for a substance use disorder."[10]

Even though the federal government contributes most of the funds, the individual states determine the eligibility guidelines for coverage. Different states have different income guidelines as to who can get Medicaid and who cannot. States were required to offer coverage for children up to at least 100 percent of FPL. Today, the average median income limit for a family of three in the twelve non-expansion states is 47.3 percent of poverty. So, a three-member family in Alabama can make no more than $75 per week in order to get Medicaid.[11] If they make slightly higher than that figure, well, there's always the emergency room—which costs taxpayers more per visit than Medicaid coverage, by the way. Heartless, stupid, and just plain mean. Go figure.

That all changed, however, in 2010 with passage of the Patient Protection and Affordable Care Act, which would provide health insurance coverage by January 2014 to all low-income citizens through Medicaid expansion, plus "Health Insurance Marketplaces," to subsidize private health insurance coverage for those who qualify at higher FPLs. Importantly, two of the ten "Essential Health Benefits" automatically covered were mental health and substance use disorder treatment and preexisting conditions.

What Is Obamacare?

To increase the number of Americans with health insurance, the federal government provides subsidies to middle-income Americans in order for them to purchase private health insurance. Additionally, by expanding Medicaid, the government makes health insurance available to more low-income Americans. Despite the baseless vitriol generated by "haters of anything Obama," "Obamacare" is *not* government insurance—it is the government helping you purchase private insurance. It is *not* a handout. It is simply one of the programs that fit into the *$1.697 trillion* the federal government spends annually subsidizing all the other health insurance programs it supports, including employer-based ones.

Government's Health Insurance Subsidies 2020 at $1.697 Trillion

Medicare (65+)	$776B[12]
Medicaid/CHIP	$433B
Work-related coverage	$303B
Medicare (under 65)	$125B
Obamacare and individuals	$60B[13]

If your annual income falls between 138 percent and 400 percent of the federal poverty level (FPL), you are eligible for help (called a Marketplace premium tax credit) from the federal government to purchase a private health insurance policy (Obamacare). It's not a "government insurance policy," but rather a policy from a company like Blue Cross or Aetna that the federal government helps you purchase. If your income falls below 138 percent of the FPL and you live in one of the thirty-six states that expanded Medicaid, you are eligible for Medicaid coverage, which the federal government pays directly to your state to provide your health insurance.

Due to the ACA and Medicaid expansion, more than twenty million Americans got health insurance coverage that they did not have before. In 2010, 48.6 million Americans lacked health insurance, and that figure declined to just below 26.5 million in the first half of 2016, which is a 20.1 million reduction per the Centers for Disease Control and Prevention. Eight million of those 20.1 million were covered by private insurance through the Marketplace Exchange (see figure 6.3).

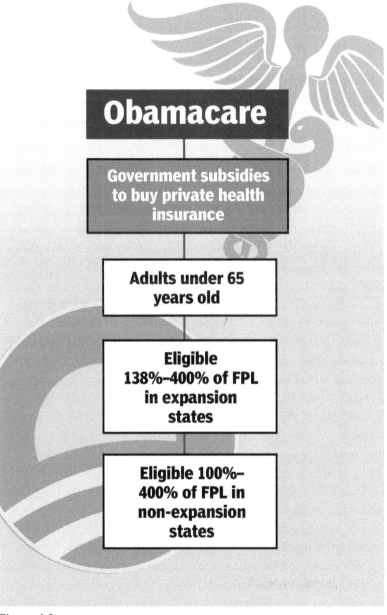

Obamacare

Government subsidies to buy private health insurance

Adults under 65 years old

Eligible 138%–400% of FPL in expansion states

Eligible 100%–400% of FPL in non-expansion states

Figure 6.3.
Source: Healthcare.gov. Art © The Right Rehab, LLC.

Unfortunately, due to the Trump administration's drive to banish the ACA, the uninsured rate climbed to thirty-two million in 2020.

The positive effects of health insurance, including behavioral health treatment, now being available to millions of citizens for whom insurance used to be out of reach were almost immediate in states that expanded their Medicaid program. Expanding the number of people with incomes below 138 percent of the federal poverty level eligible for Medicaid made it possible for those without coverage—especially single males—to finally get drug, alcohol, and mental disorder treatment.

Unfortunately, in 2012 the Supreme Court ruled that the federal government could not make Medicaid expansion mandatory for states, so several of them—primarily red states in the southern portion of the country—opted not to expand their Medicaid programs. More than nine in ten of those denied Medicaid reside in the South—nearly one-third in Texas. Seventy-six percent of those denied are adults without dependent children.[14]

Even though the federal government was covering 100 percent of an expansion state's costs from 2014 through 2018, that percentage was lowered to 93 percent in 2019 and will remain at 90 percent from 2020 onward. Despite that financial incentive, for political reasons twelve states still refused to expand their Medicaid programs—leaving at least 4.7 million otherwise eligible citizens without Medicaid coverage as of June 2020. Of those ineligible, 2.8 million of them are caught in the "coverage gap," "meaning they have incomes too high to qualify for Medicaid but too low for ACA marketplace subsidies—as well as 1.9 million more people who are at risk of losing health insurance due to job loss during the pandemic and otherwise would end up in the coverage gap."[15]

Let's see what that means if you live in one of the twelve states that did not expand Medicaid. A family of three is in the "coverage gap" and does not qualify for Medicaid if their modified adjusted gross income (MAGI) is greater than what is shown in figure 6.4.

2.8 million caught in coverage gap in non-expansion states

State	No More than % of FPL	No More than per Year	No More than per Month	No More than per Week
Alabama	18%	$3,910	$326	$75
Florida	31%	$6,733	$561	$129
Georgia	35%	$7,602	$634	$146
Kansas	38%	$8,254	$688	$159
Mississippi	26%	$5,647	$471	$109
North Carolina	41%	$8,905	$742	$171
South Carolina	67%	$14,552	$1,213	$280
South Dakota	48%	$10,426	$869	$200
Tennessee	94%	$20,417	$1,701	$393
Texas	17%	$3,692	$308	$71
Wisconsin	100%	$21,720	$1,810	$418
Wyoming	53%	$11,512	$959	$221

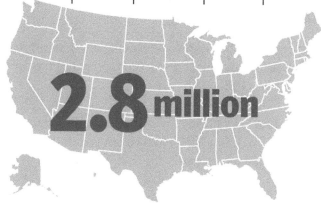

Source: Kaiser Family Foundation June 25, 2020 ©The Right Rehab, LLC

Figure 6.4.

Source: Garfield, Orgera, and Damico (2020). Art © The Right Rehab, LLC.

Between 2013 and the first half of 2018, the uninsured rate in expansion states decreased to 9.1 percent. For those that did not expand, their uninsured populations stood at 18.4 percent.[16] That's ironic for the states that thought it was in their own interest not to expand since they are "missing out on more than $305 billion in federal funding between 2013 and 2022. For residents of those states, their federal tax dollars are being used to pay for Medicaid expansion in other states, while none of the Medicaid expansion funds are coming back to their own states."[17] Furthermore, through 2022, non-expansion states will pay an additional $152 million in federal taxes for the use of Medicaid programs in expansion states.

From 2005 through 2020, hospitals in states that did not expand Medicaid saw a sharp increase of hospital closings, while states that expanded Medicaid saw closure rates decrease.[18] "Beyond the potential health consequences for the people living nearby, hospital closings can exact an economic toll, and are associated with some states' decisions not to expand Medicaid as part of the Affordable Care Act. Care for mental health and substance use are among those most likely to be in short supply after rural hospital closures."[19]

How Do I Get Marketplace or Medicaid Insurance?

To be a member of the insured population, let's first determine your modified adjusted gross income (MAGI) and percentage of the federal poverty level (FPL).

- Based on your previous year's adjusted gross income (AGI) on line 7 of Form 1040 you filed last year, estimate your AGI for the end of this year.
- Add to that figure any untaxed foreign income, nontaxable Social Security benefits (do *not* include supplemental security income—SSI), and tax-exempt interest.
- The total is your estimated MAGI.

- Looking at the FPL chart, if you have a family of four, take that annual figure and divide your MAGI by that number.
- Multiply the answer (quotient) by 100.
- That answer (product) is your family's percentage of the FPL. Example: If your estimated MAGI will be $40,000 and the annual FPL is $25,750 for a family of four, divide $40,000 by $25,750 and multiply the answer (the quotient) by 100, which equals 155.34 percent of FPL. See figure 6.5.

If You Live in an Expansion State

If you reside in a state that expanded its Medicaid program (see figure 6.6) and your FPL is between 138 percent and 400 percent of the FPL, congratulations—you are eligible for the premium tax credit that the federal government gives you to help pay for your monthly premium under the "Obamacare" program. If your income is between 100 percent and 250 percent of the FPL, congratulations again, because you are also eligible for an extra subsidy that helps pay your deductible and out-of-pocket maximum. To obtain your coverage, contact an insurance broker (his commission does not come out of your end) or Healthcare.gov at 1-800-318-2596, or you can visit the website at https://www.healthcare.gov/.

Unfortunately, unlike the "old days" when you could buy health coverage and it would begin the day of purchase, as of this writing, application for Marketplace policies must be done during the "open enrollment" period—November 1 through December 15 of the current year. Fortunately, the Biden administration extended it to August 15, 2021, due to the COVID pandemic. Coverage will begin on January 1 of the following year. However, there are exceptions called "qualifying events" within the previous sixty days:

- Loss of qualifying health insurance coverage
- Marriage
- Childbirth
- Becoming a dependent

2021 federal poverty guidelines (FPL) for the 48 contiguous states

Annual MAGI (Modified Adjusted Gross Income)

Number in household	100%	133%	138%	150%
1	$12,760	$16,971	$17,609	$19,140
2	$17,240	$22,929	$23,791	$25,860
3	$21,720	$28,888	$29,974	$32,580
4	$26,200	$34,846	$36,156	$39,300
5	$30,680	$40,804	$42,338	$46,020
6	$35,160	$46,763	$48,521	$52,740
7	$39,640	$52,721	$54,703	$59,460
8	$44,120	$58,680	$60,886	$66,180
1 (Alaska)	$15,950	$22,214	$22,011	$23,925
1 (Hawaii)	$14,680	$19,524	$20,258	$22,020

Number in household	200%	250%	300%	400%
1	$25,520	$31,900	$38,280	$51,040
2	$34,480	$43,100	$51,720	$68,960
3	$43,440	$53,340	$65,160	$86,880
4	$52,400	$65,500	$78,600	$104,800
5	$61,360	$76,700	$92,040	$122,720
6	$70,320	$87,900	$105,480	$140,640
7	$79,280	$99,100	$118,920	$158,560
8[a]	$88,240	$110,300	$132,360	$176,480
1 (Alaska)[b]	$31,900	$47,850	$47,850	$63,800
1 (Hawaii)[c]	$29,360	$44,040	$44,040	$58,720

Figure 6.5.

Source: "2021 Federal Poverty Level Chart," Kentucky Health Benefit Exchange, (2020). Art © The Right Rehab, LLC.

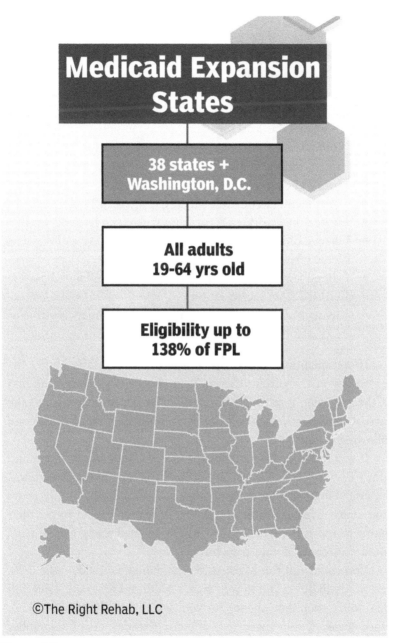

Figure 6.6.

Source: Kaiser Family Foundation. Art © The Right Rehab, LLC.

- Divorce or legal separation
- Death of someone on your plan resulting in you losing eligibility for current plan
- Change of primary residence
- New zip code or county (must have had qualifying health coverage for at least one day during the sixty days before the move, except from a foreign country or territory)
- From a foreign country
- From a shelter or transitional housing
- For students, to or from where you attend school
- For seasonal workers, to or from where you live and work
- Change of income
- Denied Medicaid or CHIP
- Gained lawful citizenship or residence in the United States
- Released from incarceration
- Member of a federally recognized Native American tribe or an Alaska Native corporation

If you qualify for a "qualifying event," by enrolling by the fifteenth day of the current month, your coverage will begin the first of the following month. If you enroll after the fifteenth day of the current month, coverage will not begin until the first of the second following month.

If you reside in a state that expanded its Medicaid program and your FPL was under 138 percent of the FPL, again, congratulations, because you are eligible for your state's Medicaid program. Contact your state's Medicaid office by calling 1-877-267-2323 to get their number or visit the website at https://www.medicaid.gov/about-us/contact-us/contact-state-page.html.

You could call the Marketplace Exchange at 1-800-318-2596, and they will direct you to your state's Medicaid program. They will also notify your state agency for you, which will then contact you. Once enrolled, your coverage is effective that day. As of September 2019, in several expansion states coverage is retroactive through the previous three months.

Sorry, You Live in a Non-expansion State

If you live in a Medicaid non-expansion state—move. But if that is not practical and your income is between 100 percent and 400 percent of the FPL, you are still eligible for a policy on the Federal Healthcare Exchange. Follow the directions in the previous section to contact the Exchange.

As of this writing, if you are an adult with dependents or you are a caretaker with an income below 100 percent FPL and living in one of the twelve states that refused to expand its Medicaid program (see figure 6.7), your options are severely limited for any substance use disorder (SUD) treatment, let alone any medical treatment other than your local emergency room. You are also one of the 4.9 million American citizens kept from receiving health insurance benefits that citizens in other states have.

There are 2.5 million uninsured adults in non-expansion states who are stuck in "the coverage gap," a purgatory above their particular state's eligibility level for Medicaid but still below 100 percent of FPL for the Federal Marketplace insurance in non-expansion states.

Where Can I Get the Treatment I Need?

If you are eligible for Medicaid, be aware that it does not cover exactly the same services in each state. If you need to know which services Medicaid covers in your state and the easiest, most efficient way to find them, go to the master list of master lists—the Substance Abuse and Mental Health Services Administration (SAMHSA) at https://www.samhsa.gov/find-treatment.

They have 15,961 treatment programs listed. If there is a program in your vicinity that fits your individual needs (including your resources), you will be able to find it in the searchable database by zip code, city, state, insurance, and treatment, among a plethora of other ways searchable information is entered. You can also call SAMHSA at 1-877-726-4727. Tell them what you need, and they will go over how to use their directory locator and point you in the right

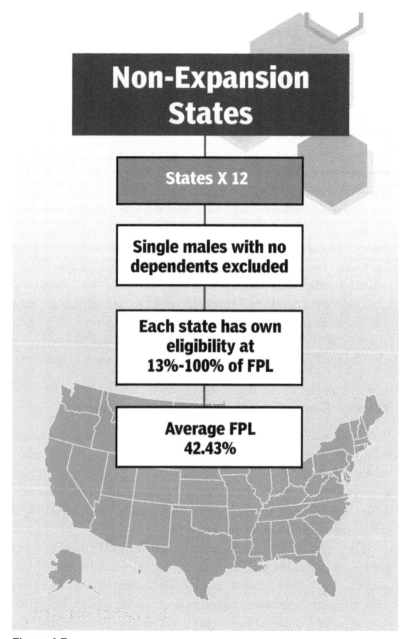

Figure 6.7.
Source: Kaiser Family Foundation. Art © The Right Rehab, LLC.

direction. SAMHSA also has a toll-free helpline staffed 24/7 and 365 days a year: 1-800-662-HELP (4357). In addition, you could get the phone number for Medicaid in your state by calling 1-877-267-2323 or visit the website at https://www.medicaid.gov/about -us/contact-us/contact-state-page.html.

If there's an immediate need for treatment, the emergency room at a local hospital should have (or at least know) a hospital that staffs a behavioral health team. When you find one, go there and ask to be diagnosed. If you are slipping into withdrawal or need to be detoxed or stabilized, they should be able to do that there or direct you to a facility that will. You will be asked for insurance, but if you are lacking insurance or cash payment and you are at a community hospital that takes Medicare and Medicaid, it is mandatory for them to attend to your immediate needs as long as you need stabilization.

Normally, they will assign a case manager who will keep track of your treatment and direct you to further treatment solutions. Case managers are key. It's their job to know local resources that can offer long-term treatment per your situation—at least, they will give you a list of them. It's also possible that a particular hospital can offer you further services—short-term or long-term residential or outpatient treatment. The point is that hospitals are in the business of knowing how to get people care, including behavioral health needs.

You could also call your local police department and ask for their crisis intervention team. Fortunately, many metropolitan police departments have officers now trained in dealing with those who are threatening suicide or harm to others. Since their job is to get treatment services to those who need it, they are familiar with the resources available in your area.

Out of the 4.2 million people who went to various forms of behavioral health treatment in 2019, the vast majority took advantage of the outpatient options available to them either exclusively or in addition to the other treatment options. "Self-help" groups such as AA (Alcoholics Anonymous) are not formally considered treatment, but rather crucial mutual support maintenance in a recovery support services (RSS) lifetime plan.

Medicare

Medicare is the federal health insurance program for people who meet certain criteria:

- People aged sixty-five or older
- People under sixty-five with disabilities and receiving Supplemental Security Income (SSI) benefits
- People with approved medical conditions—such as amyotrophic lateral sclerosis (ALS, or Lou Gehrig's disease) or end-stage renal disease (permanent kidney failure requiring dialysis or a transplant, sometimes called ESRD)—or other qualifying disabilities may also be eligible for Medicare benefits

There are four different parts to the Medicare program. Parts A and B are often referred to as Original Medicare. Medicare Part C, or Medicare Advantage, is private health insurance, while Medicare Part D offers coverage for prescription drugs.[20]

Medicare Part A is hospital insurance that covers the following:

- Inpatient hospital stays (not long-term residential drug treatment)
- Skilled nursing facility stays
- Hospice care
- Some home health care

Medicare Part B is medical insurance that covers the following:

- Doctors' services
- Outpatient care
- Medical equipment and supplies
- Home health services
- Ambulance services
- Preventative services
- Therapy services (physical, speech, occupational)

Part C is also called "Medicare Advantage" since it is offered as an alternative by private insurance companies that are paid a fixed amount per person by the federal government to provide Medicare benefits through the following:

- Health Maintenance Organizations (HMOs)
- Preferred Provider Organizations (PPOs)
- Private Fee-for-Service (PFFS)

Medicare Part D is optional prescription drug coverage offered through private companies as a stand-alone plan, but it is still a part of Medicare. You will share in the costs of your prescription drugs according to the specific plan in which you are enrolled.[21]

Medicare and Behavioral Health Treatment

Medicare covers alcoholism and SUD treatment in both outpatient and short-term inpatient settings under the following conditions:

- Your provider states that the services are medically necessary.
- You receive services from a Medicare-approved provider or facility.
- Your provider sets up your plan of care.

Covered services include, but are not limited to, the following:

- Assessment and diagnosis to determine the severity of substance use
- Brief intervention providing advice and motivation to make behavioral changes
- Referral to treatment
- Psychotherapy
- Post-hospitalization follow-up
- Prescription drugs administered during a hospital stay or injected at a doctor's office

- Methadone covered in inpatient hospital settings but not covered in outpatient clinics where it is supplied orally
- Outpatient prescription drugs covered by Part D
- Psychiatric counseling and diagnostic tests
- Individual therapy
- Group therapy
- Family counseling
- Alcohol abuse counseling (up to four sessions)
- Physician assistants
- Nurse practitioners
- General practitioners
- Clinical social workers[22]

If you receive care in a psychiatric hospital, Medicare covers up to 190 days of inpatient care in your lifetime. If you have used your lifetime days but need additional mental health care, Medicare may cover your care at a general hospital.[23]

Unfortunately, in my experience, finding facilities and psychiatrists that accept Medicare for behavioral health services is a challenge.

To find out more about services covered by Medicare, call toll-free 1-800-633-4227 or visit the website at https://www.medicare.gov/. You could also call Social Security at 1-800-772-1213 or visit the website at https://www.ssa.gov/.

Native American/Tribal Resources

"Compared to other racial/ethnic groups in the U.S., American Indians/Alaska Natives have our nation's highest rates of alcohol, marijuana, cocaine and hallucinogen use disorders and the second highest methamphetamine abuse rates after native Hawaiians. In addition, high rates of traumatic exposure have been identified among AI/ANs with alcohol use disorders."[24]

In addition, with rates higher among Native Americans than among non-Native communities—two and a half times the national average—suicide has become an epidemic in tribal nations across the country as well as substance abuse.

If you are a member of a tribe, contact your tribe's headquarters to inquire about treatment. As a tribal member or an employee of an American Native-owned company, there are likely health insurance and treatment programs available to you and your family.

You could also contact the Indian Health Service and their Alcohol and Substance Abuse Program (ASAP) by calling 1-406-745-2411.

Criminal Justice and Treatment

The United States has the highest rate in the world of people incarcerated—698 per one hundred thousand for a total of almost 2.3 million. "The American criminal justice system holds almost 2.3 million people in 1,833 state prisons, 110 federal prisons, 1,772 juvenile correctional facilities, 3,134 jails, 218 immigration detention facilities, and 80 Indian Country jails as well as military prisons, civil commitment centers, state psychiatric hospitals and prisons in U.S. territories."[25] The more than one million drug possession arrests per year are the first step for the more than five hundred thousand offenders in those facilities and contribute to the more than $181 billion it costs to hold them.

In 2018, out of the 10,310,960 arrests in our country, the offense responsible for most of them was drug abuse violations at 1,654,282, followed by DUIs at 1,001,329,678.[26]

The following are some alarming statistics (as of 2020):

- 20 percent of America's adult working population have a criminal record of some kind.
- By age twenty-three, nearly one in three Americans will have been arrested.
- As many Americans have criminal records as college diplomas.

- The United States houses roughly the same number of people with criminal records as it does four-year college graduates (see figure 6.8).
- A past criminal conviction of any sort reduced the likelihood of a job offer by 50 percent.[27]
- "More than two-thirds of jail detainees and half of prison inmates experience SUDs . . . only 10% of prison inmates receive SUD treatment services."[28]

What Is Drug Court?

> "You're learning life on life's terms and it's hard, powerful work by helping someone with addiction make the right choices knowing there is going to be accountability."
>
> —The Honorable Kenneth Stoner,
> Oklahoma County drug court judge[29]

One way to deal with the overincarceration in our country is to adjudicate nonviolent drug offenders in a separate judicial system. Drug court is that system, one that offers the drug or alcohol offender substance abuse treatment as an alternative to incarceration. By 2015, judges throughout the nation were overseeing more than thirty-four hundred drug courts to provide treatment and other services for more than fifty-five thousand offenders each year to transition back into society substance free and out of the criminal justice system.

Instead of focusing on punishment as a deterrent, all parties involved—defense attorneys, prosecutors, social workers, and judges—focus on structured programs using treatment, probation, drug testing, and eventual graduation for those who make it through the program. Their average recidivism rate is from 8 to 38 percent (depending on the region in the United States) compared to the 54 percent nationwide average recidivism rate without drug court. Thus far, drug courts have been found to reduce crime as much as 45 percent more than other sentencing options.

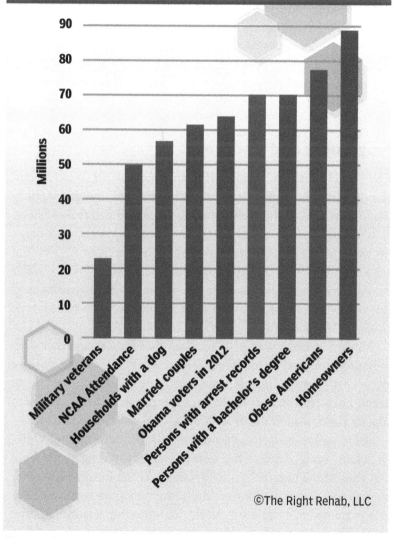

Figure 6.8.

Source: Friedman (2015). Art © The Right Rehab, LLC.

What do these figures prove? They prove that the war on drugs has had no tangible impact on crime, while treatment for substance use disorders (SUDs) has. Treatment coupled with medication-assisted therapy (MAT) has proven to be the most cost-effective way of dealing with addicted offenders afflicted with opioid-use disorders. At an average cost of $5,000 for methadone maintenance versus the average housing costs of an inmate at $30,000 per year, treatment is the better use of taxpayers' money. "For every 100 patients on methadone per year, there were 12 fewer robberies, 57 fewer break-and-enters and 56 fewer auto thefts."[30]

Drug Court and Recovery

When we compare the results of placing nonviolent, drug-related offenders in jail or prison versus placing them in treatment, drug courts provide a much better outcome for the offender and society. "A 10% relative increase in the SUD treatment rate at an average cost of $1.6 billion yields a crime reduction benefit of $2.5 billion to $4.8 billion."[31] In addition to a life in recovery, "For a dollar spent on treatment, up to three are saved in crime reduction."[32] Moreover, "an additional treatment facility reduces felony-type crimes by 10% annually."[33]

Mena Samara, owner of Bada Bing Bail Bonds, says that drug court programs "are extraordinarily successful . . . such a positive option that gives defendants hope, one more chance . . . instead of making contacts with drug dealers in jail or prison, why not give them help, let them make contacts with those who want to help them?"[34]

A former prosecutor and now a criminal defense attorney, Oklahoma City–based Ed Blau has seen the efficacy of drug courts from both ends of the criminal justice system: "As the former prosecutor assigned to Oklahoma County's drug court, and now a criminal defense practitioner, I can testify to the life-changing qualities of drug courts. They not only help participants with their sobriety, but they also help give participants a sense of pride in accomplishing something as rigorous as working through and ultimately graduating from a drug court program. Drug courts help heal the whole person."[35]

Despite being a good provider for his family, Jake saw his life shatter into a billion pieces when his wife left him—their baby daughter in tow—due to the drinking and drugs that were taking over his life. Soon, the inevitable loss of his high five-figure job deepened his whirlpool of misery, leading to his arrest for larceny and several months in the Oklahoma City jail. He jumped at the opportunity to be in the drug court program, and Jake's home for the next eighteen months became the city's Mission gymnasium shared with forty-six other men.

After losing everything but now adhering to the drug court's strict program, Jake saw his luck begin to change when he came across a still presentable pair of jeans and a button-down gingham shirt in a trash can. Finally, he had an outfit for court appearances and job interviews. Three years later, Jake is the general manager of a profitable store for a billion-dollar retail chain. Now living a life in recovery, Jake's wardrobe has expanded considerably, but it still shares the closet with the jeans and gingham shirt he rescued from that trash can.

"Although I rescued those jeans and that shirt, they really rescued me," Jake maintains. "I keep them to remind me from where I came and how far I have come."

Drug courts work. Treatment works.

CHEAT SHEET: A SUMMARY OF WHAT YOU NEED TO KNOW NOW-NOW

Chapter I Summary: Breaking the Glass

1. When in Crisis
   a. Call 911:
      i. if the individual is experiencing a psychotic episode or threatening to harm himself or someone else (ask for a crisis intervention officer to accompany responders).
      ii. if the person is unconscious from suspected overdose.
   b. If the individual is in withdrawal, take him to a hospital ER, crisis intervention center, or detox unit for stabilization.
2. When you suspect a family member or one who shares your household of being a substance user:
   a. Take a CPR course; it may be needed.
   b. Have multiple doses of Narcan available.
3. If the person is under arrest and in jail:
   a. If there is one, call the individual's defense attorney.
   b. If you need an attorney, ask those you trust for a suggestion.
   c. Using a public defender can be the best alternative.
   d. Send the person to a treatment facility right away before charges are filed or arraignment?

      i. If offense is nonviolent, the attorney should be able to clear with the district attorney and judge per the individual's criminal history.

   e. Bail

      i. Get bondsman?

      ii. Do you bond-out the person or leave in jail to stay out of trouble?

4. During this crisis, you will be asked for specific information about the individual.

   a. The more accessible the information, the smoother and more efficient the process.

   b. Refer to the list in chapter 1.

Chapter 2 Summary: What Is Treatment?

1. What Is Addiction?

   a. A chronic, long-term illness resulting from the complex interplay between one's genes and environment.

   b. Disorder of pleasure

      i. Results in the brain's inability to properly perceive pleasure.

   c. Disorder of choice

      i. Poor decisions are the result of one's malfunctioning reward system.

   d. A defect in our dopamine system caused by stress.[1]

2. What Causes Addiction?

   a. Factors include the following:

      i. Trauma caused by physical, emotional, or sexual abuse

      ii. Neglect

      iii. Family history of addiction

      iv. Parental substance use

      v. Family and peer dynamics

      vi. Household instability

      vii. Availability of drugs or alcohol

      viii. Exposure to stress

      ix. Incarceration of family members

      x. Poverty

      xi. Age when use begins

      xii. Presence of co-occurring mental disorder

      xiii. Little to no access to social support

  b. Similar to chronic diseases

      i. Hypertension

      ii. Asthma

      iii. Diabetes

3. Physical Dependence

  a. Not addiction but accompanies addiction when one's body adapts to the physical effects of a substance.

  b. Caffeine is an example of your body adapting to it, but it does not control your life as addiction does.

  c. Addiction, however, is the most severe form of substance use, associated with compulsive or uncontrolled use of one or more substances.

4. Treatment

  a. There is no cure to addiction.

  b. Treatment enables people to counteract addiction's disruptive effects on their brain and behavior to regain control of their lives.[2]

      i. A combination of behavioral therapies, medication, and recovery support services (RSS) intended as a continuum of care and lifestyle supporting long-term recovery.

  c. Key component is evidence-based therapy.

      i. Employed with goal of reaching remission leading to a lifetime of recovery.

      ii. Even after a year or two of remission is achieved through treatment, it can take three to five more years before the risk of relapse drops below 15 percent, the level of risk that people in the general population have of developing a substance use disorder (SUD) in their lifetime.[3]

5. Diagnosis
   a. In order to treat SUD, it is necessary to know exactly what needs to be treated.
   b. Must be done by a trained, certified, licensed professional.
   c. Eleven diagnostic symptoms define whether there is a disorder and its severity:
      i. Using in larger amounts or for longer than intended.
      ii. Wanting to cut down or stop using but not managing to do it.
      iii. Spending a lot of time to get, use, or recover from use.
      iv. Craving the substance.
      v. Inability to manage commitments due to use.
      vi. Continuing to use, even when it causes problems in relationships.
      vii. Giving up important activities because of use.
      viii. Continuing to use, even when it puts one in danger.
      ix. Continuing to use, even when physical or psychological problems may be made worse by use.
      x. Increasing tolerance to the substance.
      xi. Withdrawal symptoms.
6. Dual Diagnosis
   a. Also known as "co-occurring."
   b. About 40–60 percent of SUDs (substance use disorders) have an accompanying mental disorder.
   c. Most common disorders:
      i. Depression
      ii. Anxiety
      iii. Bipolar disorder
      iv. Schizophrenia
      v. PTSD
7. Primary + Secondary
   a. A professional diagnosis determines:
      i. Substance use disorder (SUD)
      ii. Mental disorder

iii. Primary SUD and secondary mental disorder

iv. Primary mental disorder and secondary SUD

8. Outpatient versus Inpatient

   a. Outpatient

      i. Treatment provides group and individual counseling in morning or evening sessions accommodating those who maintain a regular work or academic schedule.

      ii. Typically continuing care for those recently discharged from a residential program or at the initial level of care for those with mild to moderate SUDs.

   b. Three kinds of outpatient treatment that occur at a clinic:

      i. PHP (partial hospitalization programming)

      ii. IOP (intensive outpatient programming)

      iii. OP (outpatient)

   c. Inpatient

      i. Two kinds of inpatient treatment:

         (1) Medically supervised substance withdrawal delivered in an acute, inpatient hospital or dedicated medical unit—otherwise known as detox.

         (2) Thirty-day care not in a hospital, but in a hospital-like setting that offers twenty-four-hour support, staff, and structure for intensive evidence-based clinical services and therapy—otherwise known as residential.

9. Drug and alcohol treatment facilities treat addiction to substances that are primarily grouped into three major categories:

   a. Alcohol

   b. Illicit and legal drugs used illicitly

   c. Over-the-counter drugs and other substances

10. Some facilities also specialize in treating "process" addiction:

   a. Addictive behavior that does not necessarily involve substances but rather obsessive conduct that compels the individual to engage compulsively and repeatedly in behavior detrimental to the individual.

      i.   Eating disorder
      ii. Gambling
      iii. Sex and intimacy
      iv. Love
      v.   Pornography
      vi. Work
      vii. Compulsive buying/shopping
      viii. Internet
      ix. Self-harming
      x.   Codependency
      xi. Gaming

11. Mental Illness
    a. Two broad categories
       i. Not mutually exclusive
    b. Any mental illness (AMI)
       i. Includes all mental disorders
       ii. From any mental, behavioral, or emotional disorder in the past year that ranges from none to mild impairment for two weeks or less all the way up to full-blown schizophrenia
       iii. Serious mental illness (SMI)
          (1) SMI is a subset of AMI.
          (2) Adults with AMI are defined as having SMI if they had any mental, behavioral, or emotional disorder that substantially interfered with or limited one or more major life activities.
          (3) Symptoms of SMI include the inability to work, function in school, interact with family, or fulfill other major life activities.[4]

12. Evidence-Based Therapies
    a. Called "evidenced based" because of the voluminous evidence of research and studies proving that these therapies build skills to resist substance use.

b. Increases life skills to handle stressful circumstances that trigger substance use.
c. Develops coping strategies and tools to maintain abstinence:
   i. Identify the problem and be motivated to change.
   ii. Provide incentives for abstinence.
   iii. Repair damaged relationships with family and friends.
   iv. Develop personal accountability and responsibility.
   v. Build new friendships with people in recovery.
   vi. Replace substance-using activities with constructive and rewarding ones.
   vii. Improve problem-solving skills.
   viii. Create a recovery lifestyle.
d. Common therapies
   i. Cognitive behavioral therapy (CBT)
   ii. Dialectical behavioral therapy (DBT)
   iii. Matrix Model
   iv. Family behavioral therapy (FBT)
   v. Behavioral couples therapy (BCT)
   vi. Eye movement desensitization and reprocessing (EMDR); used for trauma work
   vii. Brainspotting (similar to EMDR for trauma)
   viii. Psychodrama
   ix. Medication-assisted therapy (MAT)
   x. Exposure therapy
   xi. Equine therapy
   xii. Relapse prevention
   xiii. Art therapy
   xiv. Hypnotherapy
   xv. Twelve-step programming and peer support
   xvi. Fitness
   xvii. Music therapy
   xviii. Holistic treatments
   xix. Adventure/experiential therapy

    xx. Nutritional counseling
    xxi. Life skills classes

Chapter 3 Summary: The Right Rehab

1. The "right" rehab is the one that is right for you.
  a. You need a rehab with integrity.
  b. Sources to contact:
    i. An interventionist/treatment placement specialist
      (1) Ask for multiple references.
        (a) Four at minimum.
        (b) Confirm only source of their fee is from you.
          (i) Not a referral fee from a rehab
          (ii) Confirm services with a contract
    ii. Additional sources:
      (1) Your physician
      (2) Counselors
      (3) Psychiatrists
      (4) Psychologists
      (5) Hospital behavioral health staff
      (6) Hospital ER
      (7) Someone in recovery
      (8) Your spiritual leader
      (9) Your lawyer
      (10) Families you know who you know have been affected by similar issues
      (11) Crisis intervention team at your local police department
  c. The "right rehab" is
    i. A member of NAATP.
    ii. Certified by
      (1) CARF International (Commission on Accreditation of Rehabilitation Facilities)
      (2) The Joint Commission

    iii. Licensed in the state where it is located.

    iv. The one that fits your diagnosis along with your personal and demographic factors and resources.

2. Licensure

  a. Individual's diagnosis must fit licensure of facility.

    i. Substance abuse

    ii. Mental health

    iii. Primary substance abuse, secondary mental health

    iv. Primary mental health, secondary substance abuse

    v. Primary mental health + primary substance abuse

3. Consult "Avoid the Following" in chapter 3.

4. No such thing as "the best rehab."

  a. The "best rehab" is the one that is the "best fit" for a particular individual.

  b. As there are patients with varying diagnoses, there are treatment facilities with varying programs and strengths in treating various maladies.

  c. Besides the diagnosis, there are a myriad of variables that have to fit to make a rehab the right one.

    i. Drug of choice (DOC)

    ii. Co-occurring disorder (if one is diagnosed)

    iii. Drug-related and other medical issues

    iv. Goals, milestones, and steps to achieve them

    v. Age, race, and ethnicity

    vi. Sexual orientation

    vii. Gender identity

    viii. Economic and social status

    ix. Vocation

    x. Language

    xi. Health literacy

    xii. Legal problems

    xiii. Financial and/or insurance resources

5. Do *not* . . .

  a. call toll-free numbers advertised on late-night television.

      b. pick the facility because it has the nicest website when you Google rehabs.

      c. pick a facility that cold-called you.

      d. believe the salespeople when they say they "treat everything."

          i. Those people on the other end of an 800 number are not counselors—they are salespeople in a call center after your credit card number so they can make their commission.

          (1) They'll tell you anything to get it.

6. Beware of "body brokers"

      a. They are not treatment specialists.

      b. Hang up if they offer to find you a rehab at no cost to you and a free plane ticket. (That means they are being paid by a rehab for your business.)

      c. *Stay away from them!*

7. Consult chapter 3 for a list of details of what you need to know about any rehab facility.

Chapter 4 Summary: Intervention

1. Intervention is about two things: enablement and leverage to end it.

      a. Enablement

          i. Something or somebody is enabling the individual to continue the substance use despite devastating consequences to herself, family, and friends.

          (1) Identify the source of enablement.

          (2) Plan how to cut it off.

      b. Leverage

          i. Power or influence to force change

          (1) Points of leverage:

              (a) If individual is totally dependent upon family or others, the leverage is concentrated, easy to apply, and usually results in surrender—immediately or eventually.

    (b) Could be impending loss of financial support, spouse, family, friends, home, or job if individual doesn't accept help.

    (c) The weaker the leverage, the weaker the odds of surrender.

        (i) The more independent and self-reliant the individual, the fewer the points of leverage that can be applied.

2. Prepare the intervention:

    a. If resources allow, hire a professional interventionist with excellent references.

    b. Interventionist should be the same gender as the subject of the intervention.

    c. Interventionist *must* have several facilities ready to immediately admit the patient when and if the intervention is successful.

3. Two forms of intervention (in both cases, the family unit or ones closest to individual must remain unified in cutting off the enablement to achieve the individual's surrender):

    a. CRAFT (Community Reinforcement Approach to Family Training)

      i. Family agrees that their behavior enables loved one to continue his disorder.

      ii. Instead of head-on confrontation:

        (1) Family members agree to gradually end their individual forms of enabling behavior with support and loving encouragement without emotional confrontations.

        (2) The goal is for the individual to eventually realize that he must change his life, go to treatment, or quite possibly die.

        (3) Could take days, weeks, or months.

        (4) Family must maintain unity.

          (a) It takes just one family member in a moment of weakness or sympathy to break that unity, and all effort is lost.

       (5) Danger to this form of intervention is another unexpected, outside intervention.

          (a) Injury, criminal justice issues, or, even worse, loss of life.

  b. Pack Your Shit and Go Therapy

     i. Collectively, the family unit confronts the loved one with two choices: go to this rehab now or "pack your shit and go."

     ii. Cut off the enablement now—not gradually, not later—now! Tell the individual the following:

       (1) If you go to treatment, the family is behind you and will support you every way possible.

       (2) If you don't go to treatment that we have arranged for you, any and all support from us ends immediately.

     iii. If loved one surrenders, get her to treatment as soon as possible.

       (1) Must not allow time to change her mind or the plans you have made.

       (2) If within a twelve-hour drive, go now.

       (3) If flight is necessary, leave on next flight out.

          (a) Do not let loved one out of your sight until then.

4. If family member refuses to surrender:

  a. Pack his bag and then drop him off where he wants to go.

     i. Impossibly painful for the family, but frequently the only way to make the loved one confront the devastation of his addiction head on.

5. Surrender is not guaranteed, but intervention is the final tool the family can use to change their loved one's behavior.

  a. Continued family unity in purpose and action is crucial, or the intervention will fail.

  b. Family must understand that this type of intervention can also take hours, days, weeks, or months to succeed.

Chapter 5 Summary: The Right Plan

1. Effective Treatment
   a. Can manage addiction through the right treatment, lifelong mutual support, and a self-management system that fits the individual and her resources.
      i. No one plan fits everyone.
   b. The right plan for the right someone is supported by a foundation of the following:
      i. Diagnosis
      ii. Resources
      iii. A customized treatment plan that fits the individual and resources
      iv. Adjustments when necessary
      v. Commitment to making it work
   c. Upon that foundation:
      i. Treatment has to be tailored to each person's diagnosis, drug-use patterns, and drug-related medical, mental, and social issues.
      ii. If resources allow, plan should be ninety days of evidence-based behavioral therapy, medication, and transitional living followed by an ongoing continuum of care plan of recovery support services (RSS).
      iii. The RSS must include sober living, mutual-aid support (meetings), new positive relationships, and work or continuing education in an environment supportive of a recovery lifestyle.
      iv. Individual and group outpatient sessions should continue during aftercare.
      v. If necessary, continue medication-assisted therapy (MAT), but with a plan to eventually taper off its use.
2. Resources = Recovery?
   a. Treatment ranges from a Malibu rehab for $240,000 to one that's free in a church basement.

   i. The more resources you have, the more options you have. Conversely, the fewer the resources, the fewer the options.

   ii. But do more resources guarantee recovery?

     (1) Absolutely not. Resources alone do not guarantee recovery.

     (2) It is up to the individual to achieve sobriety whether it's at a recovery version of Club Med or in a church basement.

     (3) People do live a life in recovery via twelve-step peer support and not one day of rehab.

       (a) It's just that most people need more tools that only evidence-based treatment can teach them.

3. Specialty Facility

  a. A specialty facility provides specialty substance use treatment. There are different types:

   i. Hospital (inpatient only)

   ii. Drug or alcohol rehabilitation facility (inpatient or outpatient treatment)

   iii. Mental health center

  b. Research studies and treatment experts state that anything less than ninety days of formal treatment, including medications and behavioral therapies, at a specialty facility followed by nine months of sober living and recovery support services (RSS) has limited effectiveness.

  c. Conventional ninety-day treatment regimen:

   i. Days 1 through 30: RTC (residential treatment center)

   ii. Days 31 through 60: PHP (partial hospitalization programming)

   iii. Days 61 through 90: IOP (intensive outpatient programming)

  d. Followed by nine months of sober living and RSS.

     i.   Sober living (one-year minimum; three years optimum)

    ii.   Mutual-aid support (e.g., Alcoholics Anonymous' twelve-step meetings, Narcotics Anonymous, SMART Recovery, etc.)

   iii.   Individual and group outpatient sessions

   iv.   If necessary, continue MAT, but with plan to taper off

    v.   Continued education, job, or community service

4. How to Pay for Treatment

  a. Private Pay (Cash)

     i.   Best way to ensure full ninety days of specialty treatment.

    ii.   Cost ranges from $5,000 to $80,000 per month.

   iii.   Nationwide average of $15,000 to $30,000 per month.

   iv.   Most facilities will work with you on a payment schedule.

    v.   Need for constant insurance company authorization is eliminated.

   vi.   Facility has complete control over treatment plan and execution.

   vii.   Greater ability to customize and adjust treatment plan per individual.

  viii.   Easy to extend length of stay.

   ix.   Frequently more bells and whistles for the individual's comfort and needs.

    x.   What one can afford usually determines the kind of treatment one gets.

(See figure 5.19 for a one-year treatment time line driven by private pay.)

5. Insurance

  a. Getting ninety days of treatment fully covered at specialty facility is mostly a pipedream.

     i.   Insurance authorization is required for any treatment.

      (1)   Insurance company incentivized to spend as little money as possible.

      (2)   Expense of reimbursements paid to facilities in descending order:

          (a) Detox
          (b) RTC (residential)
          (c) PHP
          (d) IOP

ii. Insurance determines medical necessity of individual's condition and length of treatment for each stage of treatment, not the facility.

iii. Regularly scheduled utilization review (UR) sessions between insurance representative and facility's clinical director are required in order to continue patient's treatment.

    (1) Could be every three, five, seven, or ten days.

iv. Based upon recent history, facilities can only estimate number of days insurance will authorize for each level of care—they are unable to guarantee the number of days.

    (1) Number of days is always determined on a case-by-case basis.

    (2) Some facilities have contracted length of stays (twenty-eight days of RTC) with insurance companies, but they are unicorns.

b. Even with insurance, patient still needs cash to cover the following:

i. Unmet deductible and out-of-pocket maximum upfront.

ii. Room and board charges when stepped down from residential to PHP.

iii. Sober living rent and living expenses.

(See figure 5.20 for a one-year treatment time line driven by insurance.)

6. Diagnosis

a. Licensure of the right facility must match the individual's diagnosis

i. Substance abuse

ii. Mental health

iii. Primary substance abuse, secondary mental health

iv. Primary mental health, secondary substance abuse

v. Primary mental disorder and primary mental health

7. Location

a. Should not be local nor relatively close to home—especially for a millennial.

   i. Avoid one that is an easy exit out the door, close to the world and people from which the individual is escaping.

   ii. Away from triggers: locations, odors, people, and such from the victim's drug life that consciously or unconsciously trigger craving for substances.

   iii. New location provides opportunity to leave past life behind and become part of a new and supportive community in recovery.

   iv. If individual is a millennial, the call parents want is "I'm not coming home" after several weeks of treatment. (This is a sign that the individual has started a new life in recovery.)

   v. For a head-of-family or employee who intends to return to place of employment, being away for thirty, forty-five, or sixty days is more likely than ninety days.

    (1) Mandatory that aftercare program is in place prior to return home from facility.

8. Intake

a. Admittance to facility is termed "intake."

b. Detailed clinical assessment and physical exam upon arrival at facility.

   i. Understanding the individual's unique physical, psychological, and behavioral nature of the substance use disorder (SUD) is needed to design optimum treatment plan.

   ii. Complete detailed history of substance misuse and mental disorders.

    (1) Age, gender, and ethnicity

    (2) Substance(s) of choice, length of use, date and amount last used

      (3) Current health issues or needs
      (4) Medical history
      (5) Family history of substance use and mental disorders
      (6) Suicide attempts or ideation
      (7) Current medications
      (8) Effects of substances on the person's life
      (9) Cultural issues around the use of alcohol or drugs
      (10) Familial relationships
      (11) Social relationships, issues, and needs
      (12) Legal or financial problems
      (13) Current living situation
      (14) Employment history, stability, problems, and needs
      (15) If relevant, school performance, problems, and needs
      (16) Any previous treatment experiences or attempts to stop substance use
      (17) What he/she wants for his/her life

c. Contraband/prohibited items check of personal items.

d. If treatment is insurance dependent, victim must meet "medical necessity" for carrier to authorize treatment.

    i.   Individual's honesty is imperative.

    ii.   Having substances in your system mandatory to meet "medical necessity," although none will overtly say you need to have "shit" in your system.

       (1) When facility says, "Don't change your behavior prior to coming to us," they're saying the patient must have substance(s) in their system prior to arrival, or else insurance is likely not to authorize residential and/or PHP levels of care.

    iii. Results of the exam are immediately relayed to the insurance company for their required authorization to start treatment.

> (1) As long as the results of the assessment fit their criteria for "medical necessity"—presence of drugs or alcohol in the system and drug history, for example—they will authorize treatment, at least for the first stage of treatment, which is usually (but not always) detox and then residential treatment.
>
> (2) If the appropriate level of substances is not present, the insurance company does not consider that person "acute" or the requested level of care—detox and/or residential—"medically necessary."

9. Detox (Detoxification)

   a. If warranted, detox is medically supervised withdrawal and stabilization in an inpatient hospital or hospital-type setting with twenty-four-hour care.

   b. At best stabilization, the purpose is to make a patient medically stable and as free as possible of substances prior to long-term treatment—with typically thirty days of residential treatment as the next stage.

   c. Typically, detox ranges from three to ten days depending upon substances in the patient's system.

   d. Many facilities place the client in detox for the first twenty-four hours for observation as a matter of course anyway.

10. RTC (Residential Treatment Center)

   a. Residential care typically takes place in a hospital-like setting for a twenty-four-hour, thirty-day, highly structured and supervised program utilizing evidence-based therapies, medication, and clinical and holistic services.

   b. The facility also provides living quarters for the patients—hence "residential."

   c. Focus is on modifying behavior through evidence-based therapies regarding substance use, resocializing through personal accountability and responsibility, and building socially productive lives.

     i. Attendance at twelve-step meetings and getting a sponsor are mandatory in most programs.

    ii. If warranted, close to half of programs in the United States introduce medication-assisted therapy (MAT) to combat craving.

  d. Insurance-dependent treatment

     i. Facility cannot guarantee number of residential days insurance company will authorize.

    ii. Be ready for carrier to step patient down to next level of care—PHP—prior to day 30 to save on payments to facility.

      (1) Facility normally keeps patient in residential setting until day 30.

        (a) In some states, the patient must be moved out of residential into off-site housing per state law when stepped down to PHP.

      (2) If patient remains in residential setting, patient doesn't realize any change in level of care.

      (3) Most facilities will charge for room and board at that point.

      (4) Insurance always has the last say regarding type and length of treatment for the individual.

11. PHP (Partial Hospitalization Programming)

  a. Conventionally begins on day 31 after thirty days of residential, but now more often begins earlier due to insurance limiting RTC coverage.

  b. Residential treatment delivered on an outpatient basis is delivered three different ways:

     i. Patient continues living and receiving residential treatment until day 30.

      (1) Facility in effect is stealing from PHP days to keep patient in residential setting.

(2) Patient is charged room and board since facility is now being reimbursed at a lower rate by the insurance company.

  ii. Treatment continues at the same residential setting, but the patient is moved to off-campus housing (sober living).

(1) Patient now pays for sober living and meals.

  iii. Treatment occurs at an off-campus clinic owned and operated by the facility or by an outside provider, while the patient moves to off-campus housing.

(1) Patient now pays for sober living and meals.

c. Sometimes called "residential lite" since it is residential treatment typically delivered on an outpatient basis.

d. Usually, a total of fifteen to twenty sessions (five sessions per week over three or four five-day weeks) for six hours per session; the number of sessions could be increased if medically necessary and the patient's progress warrants it.

e. Intended to be a milestone due to the patient leaving the cocoon of residential to live in a separate sober living environment.

  i. The first step in transitioning back into the "real world."

f. Some facilities are PHP only.

  i. Treatment and housing in two separate settings from the beginning of treatment.

  ii. Frequently, it's possible for the patient to receive six to eight weeks or more as long as insurance continues covering treatment and patient continues paying for sober living.

12. IOP (Intensive Outpatient Programming)

a. IOP is a less intensive schedule of therapy than PHP that allows the individual to integrate further into the "real world."

b. Sessions are typically group programs continuing care for those recently discharged from a residential program or at the initial level of care for those with mild to moderate SUDs.

c. Continuing to reside in sober living, the individual has a choice of morning or evening sessions at a clinic or to make time for getting a job, continuing education, or performing community service.

d. IOP fosters the patient's transition to a fully functional and active life.

e. Sessions are two or three hours each of group therapy mostly three times per week within a thirty-day window.

f. The final session of IOP usually marks the end of the ninety-day window of formal treatment.

g. The number of sessions authorized by insurance is inconsistent.

    i. The number of days to expect coverage could be less or more per the relationship between the insurance company and the facility.

    ii. Number of sessions authorized could range from twelve to twenty-four or more.

13. Aftercare

a. "Sustaining remission among those seriously affected typically requires a personal program of sustained recovery management."[5]

b. AKA Recovery Support Services (RSS)

    i. Nine-month balance of one-year treatment plan.

    ii. Continuing care to help set individual up with a foundation of maintaining sobriety, preventing relapse, and living a lifetime in recovery.

    iii. Encourage starting new, sober life locally or location other than hometown, especially for millennials.

c. Services built around providing all levels of social and therapeutic services designed to support long-term self-management:

i. Outpatient Programming (OP)
   (1) One hour per week of group therapy

ii. Private sessions with a psychologist or licensed counselor when needed

iii. Continued living in sober living environment
   (1) One-year minimum
   (2) Three years optimum

iv. Mutual support groups, including consistent attendance at twelve-step or other peer support groups

v. Career and job counseling

vi. Employment or job training

vii. Life skills training

viii. Financial, budget, and banking counseling

ix. Continued education

x. Healthy nutrition

xi. Transportation availability

xii. Legal assistance

xiii. Community service

xiv. Fitness

xv. Childcare resources

14. Sober Living
  a. Provides both a substance-free environment and mutual support from fellow residents.
  b. Ideally starting with the outpatient treatment stage of formal treatment, sober living at a minimum should last the balance of the one-year treatment plan—the final nine months after formal treatment.
  c. Statistics show that those who stay in sober living for at least one year have a much higher rate of maintaining sobriety than those who don't; sobriety rates are even higher if the stay is three years.
  d. Sober living house principles should be:
    i. Random drug-testing
    ii. Random contraband search

    iii. Working at a job, looking for a job, continuing education, or community service is mandatory

    iv. Twelve-step or other peer support group meeting attendance is mandatory

    v. Curfew

    vi. Spending the night out of the housing is a privilege earned

    vii. Allow MAT?

    viii. When rules are broken:

        (1) Immediate expulsion or offer second chance

15. Medication-Assisted Therapy (MAT)

    a. Controversial in some circles but a lifesaver in others.

    b. MAT is medication used by those in treatment and recovery to counter cravings for illicit substances.

       i. The cycle of euphoria, crash, and craving—sometimes repeated several times a day—is hallmark of addiction.

       ii. In contrast, methadone and buprenorphine have gradual onsets of action and produce stable levels of the drug in the brain.

       iii. As a result, patients maintained on these medications do not experience a rush, while they also markedly reduce their desire to use opioids.[6]

    c. Not to be used alone, but simultaneously, with evidence-based therapy.

       i. Proven to produce higher rates of remission.

       ii. Reduces the rates of relapse, cravings, and risk of death due to overdose.

       iii. Reduces injection drug use and HIV transmission.

    d. Contrary to the abstinence-only ethos.

       i. MAT has critics since some of the medications used are opioids themselves.

    e. Out of 15,961 treatment programs surveyed by SAMHSA, just 7,770 (48.7 percent) use any form of MAT.[7]

    f. Medications used for opioid addiction include the following:

       i. Methadone

      ii. Buprenorphine

    iii. Naltrexone (Vivitrol)

  g. Medications used for alcohol addiction include the following:

       i. Disulfiram

      ii. Acamprosate

    iii. Naltrexone (Vivitrol)

16. Mutual-Aid Support Groups

  a. "50% of those who started attending AA meetings after formal treatment are still participating in meetings 3 years later."[8]

  b. Sometimes mistaken for treatment, twelve-step self-help groups such as AA's (Alcoholics Anonymous) mutual support are essential to most of those in recovery.

       i. Although, there are those in recovery who did not go to treatment and credit AA meetings for their sobriety.

  c. Built on two principles:

       i. A twelve-step plan of action.

      ii. The existence of a higher power than oneself.

  d. Its mutual support is based on *members sharing a problem, and through experiential knowledge and peer support, they learn from each other and focus on personal-change goals.*

  e. Al-Anon is a mutual support group for families that fosters emotional stability and encourages "loving detachment" from the afflicted loved one rather than insisting they get into treatment.

       i. Eighty percent of Al-Anon members happen to be female.

  f. Benefits of participation in AA and NA include the following:

       i. Lower health care costs associated with relapses.

      ii. Helps members cope with awkward social situations, depression, and craving.

        iii.   Offers support from other members in getting through difficult times when one's reaction was once to use substances.

17. The family must also be in recovery.
   a. Most often, a family member goes to treatment, and when he returns, the family expects him to be "fixed." However, the family has to be "fixed" as well.
      i. The family must also be in recovery.
      ii. One's addiction and/or mental disorder is frequently a manifestation of what's going on at home.
   b. When in treatment, facility therapist must run family therapy sessions with the patient and family members at least once per week in person or via video link.
      i. The family must be encouraged to seek therapy on its own as well.
   c. Only when the family unit owns its role in the recovery process will the individual and the family be on a path to recovery. You can't have one without the other.
   d. Get the book that is universally acclaimed as the best one on this subject: *It Takes a Family* by Debra Jay.

18. Relapse (the return to alcohol or drug use after a significant period of abstinence[9])
   a. Relapse is likely since recurrence rates are similar to other chronic diseases.
   b. More than 60 percent of people treated for substance use disorder (SUD) relapse within the first year of discharge from treatment and remain at increased risk of relapse for many years.[10]
   c. Relapse doesn't mean treatment was a failure—far from it.
   d. Relapse indicates that whatever was working before is not working now. It's time for adjustments.
   e. Steps to follow after relapse include the following:
      i. The individual's total dedication to sobriety and eventual recovery has to be priority one.

ii. If necessary, reinstate treatment, but with adjustments based upon what's known now.

iii. Consider instituting medication-assisted therapy (MAT) if not already being used.

iv. Tweak the recovery support services (RSS) based on what was working before.

v. Is the individual living in an environment conducive to a lifestyle of recovery?

f. It's not an anomaly for victims to go through multiple treatment programs before they finally "get it."

g. "It's one thing to know the tools, but sometimes you need help remembering how to use them."

Chapter 6 Summary: How to Get Treatment

1. Treatment for substance use disorder (SUD) and mental illness is the new battleground between the "haves" and the "have-nots."

   a. In 2020, 61.2 million of us eighteen or older had either SUD or mental illness—9.5 million had both.

   b. Of the 20.4 million people who needed SUD treatment, only 4.2 million actually received it.

   c. Of the 51.7 million with a mental illness—just more than 20 percent of our fellow citizens—more than half (28.7 million) did *not* get treatment.

2. The majority of those who wanted treatment did not receive it due to the following:

   a. Lack of funds for private pay

   b. Lack of health insurance

   c. Lack of funds for those who have insurance but are under-insured

3. Even employer-based insurance does not guarantee an individual getting treatment.

   a. 122 million in our country received employer-sponsored health insurance.

b. 30.5 million of them are underinsured and cannot afford to use it due to ever-increasing deductibles, out-of-pocket maximums, and employee share of premiums that have consistently outpaced any wage increases.

4. Despite formidable barriers, there are ways to get treatment.

   a. There are several types of payment accepted by those 15,961 facilities surveyed by SAMHSA.

5. Medicaid and Medicare are government-funded and supervised programs that serve two groups of Americans needing assistance in getting crucial health care that otherwise would not be available.

   a. Medicaid is a federal/state partnership providing health care coverage for low-income families.

      i. It is the primary health insurance coverage for close to seventy-four million low-income Americans between the ages of nineteen and sixty-four years old.

      ii. Medicaid, however, before expansion did not cover adults without dependent children. That's still a problem in the non-expansion states since among uninsured adults (especially young adult males), 12 percent have an active SUD.

   b. Medicare is a federal program providing health coverage for more than sixty-one million Americans aged sixty-five and older, as well as for those under sixty-five and disabled.

6. What is the Affordable Care Act (Obamacare)?

   a. To increase the number of Americans with health insurance, the federal government provides subsidies to middle-income Americans in order for them to purchase private health insurance; plus, by expanding Medicaid, it makes health insurance available to more low-income Americans as well, including adults without children.

   b. Despite the baseless vitriol, "Obamacare" is *not* government insurance—it is the government helping you purchase *private* insurance.

c. It is *not* a handout. It is simply one program that fits into the $1.697 trillion the federal government spends annually subsidizing all the other health insurance programs, including employer-based ones.

7. Which government programs am I eligible for if I am under sixty-five?

   a. The first step is to determine a family's household income.

8. How do I determine my family's income?

   a. The Federal Poverty Level (FPL) is "a measure of [household] income" issued every year by the Department of Health and Human Services (HHS) that is used to determine your eligibility for certain programs and benefits.

   b. Based upon your previous year's adjusted gross income (AGI) on line 7 of Form 1040 you filed last year, estimate your expected AGI for the end of this year.

      i. Take your estimated AGI and add any untaxed foreign income, nontaxable Social Security benefits (do *not* include supplemental security income—SSI), and tax-exempt interest. That total is referred to as your modified adjusted gross income (MAGI).

      ii. Looking at the FPL chart (figure 6.5), if you are a family of four, for example, take that annual figure and divide your MAGI by that number.

      iii. Multiply the answer (quotient) by 100.

      iv. That answer (product) is your family's percentage of the FPL.

      v. Example: If your estimated MAGI will be $40,000 and the annual FPL is $25,750 for a family of four, divide $40,000 by $25,750 and multiply the answer (the quotient) by 100, which equals 155.34 percent of FPL. This means your household income is 155.34 percent of the federal poverty level (FPL).

9. If you live in a state that expanded Medicaid:

   a. If your household income is between 138 percent and 400 percent of the FPL (see figure 6.5) . . .

        i.   You are eligible for the premium tax credit that the federal government gives you to help pay for your monthly premium.

    b. If your income is between 100 percent and 250 percent of the FPL . . .

        i.   You are also eligible for an extra subsidy that helps pay your deductible and out-of-pocket maximum.

    c. To obtain your coverage, contact Healthcare.gov at 1-800-318-2596 or visit the website at https://www.healthcare.gov/.

10. If you live in a state that expanded Medicaid:

    a. If your annual income falls under 138 percent of the FPL (see figure 6.5) . . .

        i.   You are eligible for your state's Medicaid program.

        ii.   Contact your state's Medicaid office by calling 1-877-267-2323 to get its number or visit the website at https://www.medicaid.gov/about-us/contact-us/contact-state-page.html.

        iii. You could also call the Marketplace Exchange at 1-800-318-2596, and they will direct you to your state's Medicaid program. They will also notify your state agency for you, which will then contact you.

11. If you reside in one of the twelve states that *did not* expand Medicaid . . .

    a. If your income is between 100 percent and 400 percent of the FPL, you are still eligible for a policy on the Federal Marketplace Exchange.

    b. As of this writing, twelve states have refused to expand Medicaid, keeping 4.9 million American citizens from receiving health insurance benefits that people in other states have.

    c. 2.5 million of those uninsured adults in non-expansion states are stuck in "the coverage gap," a purgatory above their particular state's eligibility level for Medicaid but still below 100 percent of FPL for the Federal Marketplace insurance in non-expansion states.

    d. If you are an adult with dependents or are a caretaker for one who is disabled and living in a non-expansion state with an income below 100 percent, your options for SUD treatment are severely limited to nonexistent.

12. Contact numbers and links for instructions and eligibility qualifications for Medicaid or the Insurance Marketplace (Obamacare):

    a. https://www.healthcare.gov/income-and-household-information/how-to-report/

OR

    b. https://www.healthcare.gov/income-and-household-information/how-to-report/#dontknowAGI

    c. For help to determine your income if you are unemployed:

      i. https://www.healthcare.gov/unemployed/coverage/#unemployedincune

    d. For help to determine your income if you are self-employed:

      i. https://www.healthcare.gov/self-employed/income/

13. There are four different parts to the Medicare program.

    a. Both Parts A and B are often referred to as Original Medicare.

    b. Part A is hospital insurance.

      i. Covers 80 percent of those costs.

      ii. Remaining 20 percent of costs are the patient's responsibility and can be covered by private insurance.

    c. Part B covers physician and care-related services such as doctor visits, outpatient care, and deductibles.

    d. Part C is private health insurance that is also called Medicare Advantage.

    e. Part D covers for prescription drugs.

14. Medicare and Behavioral Health

    a. Covers SUD treatment as outpatient and short-term inpatient—such as detox and acute stabilization.

    b. Finding long-term residential/inpatient care is a challenge.

   c. Majority of Medicare-related care is in a hospital or in a hospital-related facility.

   d. To find out more about services covered by Medicare, call toll-free 1-800-633-4227 or visit https://www.medicare.gov/.

   e. You could also contact Social Security at https://www.ssa.gov/ or call 1-800-772-1213.

15. Criminal Justice and Treatment

   a. More than thirty-four hundred drug courts throughout the country.

   b. Purpose is to adjudicate nonviolent drug offenders in a separate judicial system that offers SUD treatment instead of focusing on punishment.

   c. Average recidivism rate is between 8 percent and 38 percent per region compared to the national average of 54 percent without drug court.

   d. Drug courts thus far have reduced crime by 45 percent more than other sentencing options.

16. Native American/Tribal Resources

   a. Rates of suicide and substance abuse are higher in Native American communities than anywhere else in our nation.

   b. If you are a member of a tribe, contact your tribe's headquarters to inquire about treatment.

   c. If you are an employee of an American Native-owned company, there are likely health insurance and treatment programs available to you and your family.

   d. Contact the Indian Health Service and their Alcohol and Substance Abuse Program (ASAP) by calling 1-406-745-2411.

AFTERMATH: WHAT WE NEED TO DO

This may be the final chapter of this book, but the final chapter on mass addiction and death has yet to be written. We know how the first two epidemics of mass addiction eventually came to an end: the first by a federal crackdown; the second through programs educating our nation that addiction is a disease and a call to arms for government-sponsored treatment programs. When and how this current wave will end is not known.

We also know that our get-tough "wars on drugs" have been failures with only mass incarceration and shattered lives to show for them.

This third wave of mass addiction will end only when met on an equally mass scale with preventative intervention, education, full integration of mainstream medicine and behavioral health, and most of all, treatment for all those who need and want it.

Who Goes to Treatment?

Not enough who need it.

In 2019, more than twenty million people aged twelve or older (that's one in thirteen or 7.8 percent) needed substance use disorder (SUD) treatment. An estimated 2.6 million (13 percent) of them actually received treatment at a specialty facility, or what we normally would call rehab—inpatient and/or outpatient treatment.[1] What about the remaining 17.8 million? Why didn't they get treatment? The primary reasons were "no health care coverage and could not afford the cost." "Under current law, nearly half (45%) of the remaining uninsured are outside the reach of the ACA either because their state did not expand Medicaid, they are subject to immigrant eligibility restrictions, or their income makes them ineligible for financial assistance."[2] Now, that's a problem, and we can do something about it. Other reasons for not going to treatment include the following:

- *Not ready to stop using.* Unfortunately, you can't make someone get and stay sober. The person may know she has SUD, but she has to want to get sober in order to do it. Unless and until there's an intentional or unintentional intervention such as convincing by a loved one, criminal justice issues, loss or impending loss of a job, or loss of friends, family, housing, job, and money—otherwise known as "hitting bottom"—getting sober is completely up to the individual.

- *Might have negative effect on job.* The stigma that addiction (or a mental illness) results from a moral failing or a person's bad character still persists, which makes it difficult for others to recognize addiction for what it really is—a chronic brain disease that is treatable and manageable. If you keep on drinking or drugging, chances are you're going to lose your job anyway—or at worst cause a fatal injury—so why not do something about it now? In fact, treatment that is supported by an employer produces higher remission rates than treatment supported by friends and family. Enlightened employers know that an employee in recovery is most often their most productive and reliable one.

- *Might cause neighbors or community to have a negative opinion.* Guess what? They already do and wish you would do something about it.

- *Did not know where to go for treatment and did not find a program that offered the preferred type of treatment.* That's a lame excuse for not going to treatment. With more than 15,000 treatment programs recognized by the Substance Abuse and Mental Health Services Administration (SAMHSA), there's one out there that fits you. First, you should have a diagnosis from a certified, licensed caregiver. It does take work, but the right facility that's the right fit for you or a loved one and the diagnosis is out there. You just have to know what and who to ask.
- *Concerned about confidentiality.* With today's HIPPA rules, physicians, caregivers, therapists, counselors, or hospitals are prohibited under stiff penalties from releasing any information—including even being aware of the patient—unless consent has been given by the patient to release information to certain individuals. So, that excuse doesn't hold water.

In addition, roughly half of those making an appointment for treatment do not appear for their first appointment, and another 20 percent or more fail to appear for the second appointment.[3] The ones who more readily follow through going to treatment are those whose treatment is motivated by an employer, incarceration, or the threat "it's living under a bridge for you." Those more likely to go are women and people lucky enough to have a medical insurance policy. Unfortunately, those who are older and have lived with a severe and chronic addiction over an extended amount of time tend to eschew treatment altogether.

The Net Benefits of Treatment

When I was a young boy, my first trip to New York City was like going to Oz. Never had I seen anything like that city's mass of energy on its streets and sidewalks. At that time in the 1960s, it was common to see street hustlers enticing tourists to bet on "sure win" games like the "three shell game." The hustler would hide a pea under one of three walnut shells and shuffle them around on a small board. When he stopped, you'd guess under which shell the pea was hiding.

All you have to do is not take your eye off the shell hiding the pea so when he stops moving them around, you know the right one. Easy money, right? Wrong. No matter how many times you play, never, ever will you win. The house always wins.

For me, that shell game is analogous to treatment—but with better odds for the patient. Fortunately, there is quantifiable evidence that treatment for drug and alcohol addiction works for the individual and returns a positive monetary gain for society. Is it guaranteed to work every time? No. When you're dealing with human beings, there's an infinite number of variables; however, it always comes down to the commitment of the person to make it work. Knowing that, unless and until something better comes along, prevention and evidence-based treatment are the sharpest and most effective arrows in our quiver.

> Policy makers are generally more inclined to support treatment programs if they "pay for themselves" through reductions in other types of costs, e.g., health care, criminal justice costs, etc. On average, substance abuse treatment costs are associated with a monetary benefit to society representing a 7:1 ratio of benefits-to-cost primarily because of reduced costs of crime and increased employment earnings.[4]

Take, for instance, a treatment study published in 2006, the Benefit-Cost in the California Treatment Outcome Project, funded by the California Department of Alcohol and Drug Programs (ADP) and by the Robert Wood Johnson Foundation.[5] The study states that substance abuse treatment "is associated with a societal benefit representing a 7:1 ratio of benefits to costs (9:1 when arrest data are 'inflated' to proxy for actual crimes committed). 65% of the total benefit was attributable to reduction in crime costs, including incarceration. 29% was because of increased employment earnings, with the remaining 6% because of reduced medical and behavioral health costs."[6]

Taking several variables into account, this study has been quoted for several years as proof that treatment can return positive net benefits for the individual, the family, and society as a whole.

The National Institute on Drug Abuse (NIDA) states the following regarding drug treatment:

- Treatment is less expensive than not treating or incarceration (one-year methadone maintenance = $7,000 versus $35,000[7] for imprisonment).
- Every $1 invested in treatment yields $7–$9 in net benefits due to reduced crime-related costs.
- Savings can exceed costs by twelve to one when health care costs are included.
- Treatment reduces drug use by 40–60 percent.
- Treatment decreases criminal activity during and after treatment.
- Treatment reduces the risk of HIV/AIDS.
- People see employment gains of 40 percent after treatment.
- People who sought treatment saw reduced interpersonal conflicts, improved productivity, and fewer drug-related accidents.[8]

How They Do It in Washington State

Need more proof? In the state of Washington, there is a nonprofit research group—the Washington State Institute for Public Policy—whose goal is to "carry-out practical, non-partisan research at legislative direction on issues of importance to Washington State." Spanning multiple areas of responsibility for the state of Washington's governing body, the institute's mission is to find "what works and what does not in public policy."[9] Determining the best way to fight substance abuse is one of them.

If there's ever a program that should be an archetype for every state to follow in fighting the current drug and alcohol addiction epidemic, this is it. In search of "benefit-cost results," the institute's mantra is to use "evidence-based policies" that lead to programs "that can, with a high degree of certainty, lead to better statewide outcomes coupled with a more efficient use of taxpayer dollars."[10]

Using evidence-based tools and persistent follow-up with the individual, Washington State has developed programs that accurately quantify addiction treatment's cost-to-benefit. And the studies are continuous, in real time, and always being updated.

For those who do not think treatment is the answer to substance use and mental disorders, table 8.1 proves you wrong.[11]

Table 8.1. Substance Use Disorder (SUD) Treatment for Adults

Program	Benefits Minus Costs	Benefit-to-Cost Ratio	Chance Benefits Greater Than Costs
Intervention in primary care	$19,989	$1: $35.41	77%
Intervention in hospital	$2,248	$1: $14.75	70%
Contingency management	$19,989	$1: $34.41	78%
Cognitive behavioral skills	$5,755	$1: $22.31	56%
Marijuana dependence	$7,788	$1: $14.74	91%
Sober living houses	$1,135	$1: $4.89	52%
Methadone maintenance	$4,899	$1: $2.28	89%
Buprenorphine maintenance	$3,778	$1: $1.81	88%

"Benefit-Cost Results," Washington State Institute for Public Policy, http://www.wsipp.wa.gov/BenefitCost?topicId=7.

The Benefits of the Affordable Care Act (ACA) and Medicaid Expansion

"Not unlike 'voter suppression,' a powerful political force in our country is behind 'insurance suppression.'"

—Walter Wolf

"The number of uninsured nonelderly individuals dropped from more than 46.5 million in 2010 to fewer than 26.7 million in 2016."[12] "The share of Americans without medical insurance fell steadily since 2014 but then leveled off in 2016, the year Donald Trump became President."[13] These studies mark the first time since enactment of the ACA that the number of uninsured has increased, signaling that the damage President Donald Trump and his faithful followers meant to inflict on President Obama's signature accomplishment is taking effect. Eventually, with the additional one million who lost their employer-sponsored insurance along with their jobs due to the pandemic, "the number of people without health insurance is projected to rise from 32 million in 2020 to 35 million in 2029."[14]

From cutting 90 percent of funding for programs that guided the public in enrolling in the Marketplace and Medicaid to scrapping the individual mandate that helped insurance companies absorb the preexisting coverage requirement, to establishing "public charge" rules that makes it easier for immigration officials to deny visas to immigrants who use Medicaid, to establishing work requirements for Medicaid coverage meant to confound people with bureaucratic red tape, people are losing health coverage as intended by those driven by hatred for anything Obama.

> "A lot of people don't like the Affordable Care Act; they've never liked it and anything that's emanated from it is by definition 'evil' and people will look for any reason to besmirch it."
>
> —Dr. Lee Norman, Kansas secretary of health, 2019[15]

"The Census data are clear—the uninsured rate for kids is up sharply and it's due to a loss of public coverage—mostly Medicaid," Joan Alker, executive director of Georgetown University Center for Children and Families, said in a statement. "This serious erosion of children's health coverage is due in large part to the Trump Administration's actions that have made health care harder to access and have deterred families from enrolling their children."[16]

In fact, Medicaid expansion has "saved the lives of at least 19,200 adults aged 55 to 64 over the four-year period from 2014 to 2017.

Conversely, 15,600 older adults died prematurely because of state decisions not to expand Medicaid. The life-saving impacts of Medicaid expansion are large: an estimated 39% to 64% reduction in annual mortality rates for older adults gaining coverage."[17] See figure 8.1.

Additionally, for those who insist that the uninsured will always have medical care when they need it via a hospital's emergency room—well, guess what? We all pay for it. "Uncompensated care costs" are what hospitals call costs they endure when not compensated through cash or insurance by a patient who received their medical services. Usually emergency room charges, they are also typically the most expensive care one can receive.

According to the American Hospital Association (AHA), hospitals were stiffed $46.8 billion in 2013, but by 2017, that figure was $38.4 billion. Why the difference? The answer: the Affordable Care Act (the ACA, otherwise known as Obamacare) and its Medicaid expansion.

"Medicaid expansion resulted in increases in the shares of people with a personal physician, getting check-ups and getting recommended preventive care such as cholesterol and cancer screenings and decreases in the shares of people delaying care due to costs, skipping medications due to costs or relying on the ER for care, studies have found."[18]

One newly insured individual joins millions of other insured individuals, and pretty soon a lot of good stuff happens:

- Dramatic declines in infant and child mortality
- Reduced teen mortality
- Improved long-run educational attainment
- Reduced disability
- Lower rates of hospitalization and emergency department visits later in life
- Increased tax collections due to higher earnings in adulthood
- Increased access to mainstream care and behavioral health treatment

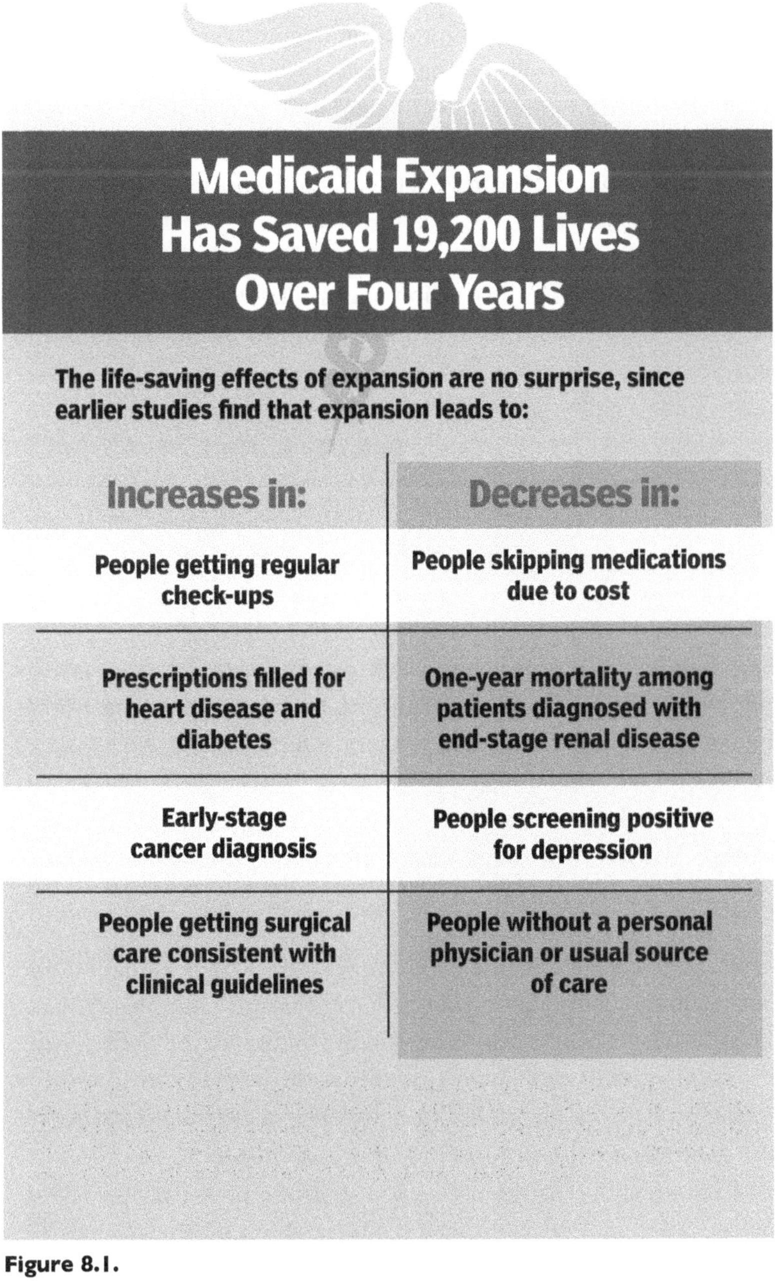

Medicaid Expansion Has Saved 19,200 Lives Over Four Years

The life-saving effects of expansion are no surprise, since earlier studies find that expansion leads to:

Increases in:	Decreases in:
People getting regular check-ups	People skipping medications due to cost
Prescriptions filled for heart disease and diabetes	One-year mortality among patients diagnosed with end-stage renal disease
Early-stage cancer diagnosis	People screening positive for depression
People getting surgical care consistent with clinical guidelines	People without a personal physician or usual source of care

Figure 8.1.

Source: Broaddus and Aron-Dine (2019). Art © The Right Rehab, LLC.

- Increased access to improved self-reported health
- Reduced mortality among adults
- Reduced financial strain on community, nonprofit, and rural hospitals
- Less public money needed to cover uncompensated care costs[19]

Multiple studies of the ACA have found larger declines in trouble paying medical bills in expansion states relative to non-expansion states and significant reduction in the number of unpaid bills and debt sent to third-party collection agencies.[20]

Whichever the number, Medicaid expansion reduced the number of bills that went into collection status, which has resulted in better credit scores and lower mortgages for auto and consumer loans. The now-insured individual and family's gain of an average $280 per year on interest payments led to $520 million available across the expansion states for consumer spending or savings. "Access to health insurance and a reduction in medical expenses has the potential to improve access to credit markets, increase savings and facilitate consumption of other goods and services. These other channels can potentially have salutary effects on the wellbeing of low-income individuals."[21]

I believe the technical term for this is "Hey, we're really kicking ass here." Economists call it a direct link between medical insurance and economic stimulation.

You're probably thinking, "Hey, Wolf, I thought this was a book about getting treatment for drug and alcohol addiction and mental illness. Why the lecture about Medicaid?" Simple. Want to get treatment? Unless you have several thousands of dollars lying around, despite its problems, insurance is the best way to access that treatment. By expanding Medicaid, we expand the number of people who get behavioral health treatment. It's no mystery.

Like waving a bright red cape in front of a deranged two-thousand-pound bull, nothing gets conservative politicians and TV pundits angrier than Obamacare. Personally, I have witnessed how health insurance through Healthcare.gov made the difference in allowing desperate families and individuals to receive badly needed SUD treatment.

Early in my service, I would frequently see people of all ages who needed treatment for SUDs and/or mental health, but the lack of health insurance kept them away from the treatment. Once I determined the facility that was the right fit for them, together we would call the Marketplace 800 number. Within one hour, they would have coverage—most often for the first time in their lives—and actual treatment waiting for them. Experiencing the tearful relief of a thirty-something mother of three is humbling.

Despite the expansion of Medicaid, however, there still are uncompensated care costs, albeit lower than before the ACA. Around 65 percent of those costs are usually covered by "practitioners and institutions, both public and private; the federal government, localities and states that support the operation of hospitals and clinics; and philanthropic donations."[22]

Several hospitals still try to collect from the patient. The result all too often is the patient getting billed a much higher amount than a patient with insurance since there is no insurance carrier negotiating the price. When the patient is unable to pay, the bill is sent to a collection agency, the patient's credit record is ruined, and the patient has now doubled his chances of filing for bankruptcy over the next four years. "Uninsured individuals who become hospitalized experience a host of financial setbacks over the next four years including reduced access to credit, a 170% increase in unpaid medical bills and a more than doubling in the likelihood of filing for bankruptcy."[23] You're welcome.

You Want *How Much* for That Box of Tissues?

Ever wonder how a hospital could charge an insane amount of money for something ordinary, like $100 for a box of tissues, and expect payment? Don't take it from me—believe Stanley F. Hupfeld, former CEO and president of Integris Health, Oklahoma's largest hospital system, which is also one of the largest hospital systems in the nation. How many hospital executives do you know who have a charter school named after them? That alone should tell you about Stan's character. In my book (literally), he knows more about health care than anybody else on this planet.

Hupfeld explains one way hospitals make up their uncompensated care costs in his recent book, *Political Malpractice: How the Politicians Made a Mess of Health Reform.* "In most industrialized nations, this source of payment is the government using tax dollars. In the United States, this source is the holders of health insurance policies." Since hospitals pass along these costs when negotiating rates of reimbursement with insurance providers, "the insurers, in turn, then build that cost into their premium structure.

"So, while the rest of the world supports care for the poor through tax dollars, we do it through our premium payments. Some part of every medical bill, whether as part of our private portion or part of the premium dollar, is financing the expense of this cost shift."[24]

In other words, for all those who are unable to pay or those who refuse to pay, the rest of us collectively underwrite their emergency room visits—the most expensive care available—and subsequent medical care anyway. Wouldn't it make more sense to put them on Medicaid, a less expensive and more efficient way of providing health coverage to those who need it?

"Healthcare does not fit into the schema of a free-market economy. In a free market, if you show up to a car dealership with the intention to drive away with a new Cadillac, you simply cannot do it without paying, short of robbery. With medical care, that is simply not the case. If you show up at an emergency room in need of care, you will not be turned away. This is an economy in which, regardless of intent, we all share the risk."[25] The question is: Are some people paying more than their fair share, and are they getting the care for what they are paying?

When it comes to sharing a great deal of that risk, rural hospitals are getting kicked in the teeth. "Nearly 1 in 5 Americans live in rural areas and depend on their local hospital for care."[26] Since January 2005, 176 of them have closed. Between 2014 and 2020, sixty rural hospitals shut their doors. Forty-eight (or 80 percent) of them were in non-expansion states, predominantly in the southern United States.[27]

Primarily in "red" states throughout the southern United States, closures of rural hospitals inflict ancillary economic damage throughout and beyond the community itself. "Beyond the potential health consequences for the people living nearby, hospital closings can exact an economic toll, and are associated with some states' decisions not to expand Medicaid as part of the Affordable Care Act. Care for mental health and substance use is among those most likely to be in short supply after rural hospital closures."[28]

Sara Barry, CEO of the Oklahoma City Primary Care Association, is a leader fighting the battle between the bedrock of our nation's health care—community health centers and other safety-net providers such as rural hospitals—and uncompensated care costs. "Individuals with untreated mental health and addictive disorders are dying an average twenty-five years before those without these conditions or those with access to care. Without question, access to necessary care is a matter of life or death. Medicaid expansion provides people that ability to get help before 'their house has burned to the ground.'"[29]

Those state representatives who continue to block Medicaid expansion and then attach work requirements in order to get it have been remarkably successful in fooling their voters to stay sufficiently uninformed and ill informed in order to continue voting against their own self-interests. I cringe each time I hear someone rant, "Why should I give my hard-earned money to those who don't deserve it?"

The hypocrisy is staggering. For those who resent paying for "freeloaders," they are completely clueless that they are paying for them anyway with the check they write every month for overpriced insurance premiums. Plus, they are paying Cadillac prices for something that should be the cost of a motor bike.

What to Do Now-Now

If it were up to me, the following is the prescription for a healthier population and continued economic expansion:

- To build and maintain an economically healthy nation, we must first have healthy citizens who then become healthy taxpayers and contributors to our nation. We have a tool that is the closest to a silver bullet in ridding us of the trillion dollars plus pound of flesh that addiction and mental illness rip from our nation's citizens each and every year—it's called treatment.

  The best way to get treatment is through health insurance. The best way to provide insurance is by expanding the ACA and Medicaid for every adult citizen and without work requirements that have proven to take insurance away from those who need it and do nothing to increase employment.

- Opposition lawmakers need to stop chipping away at the ACA. Thirty million people who didn't have health insurance in the past have it today thanks to the ACA—thirty-two million are now without it. Unless and until a better plan comes along, those who oppose it must stop trying to kill it.

- End the discrimination and punishment against those who do not qualify for Medicaid only because they do not meet the unrealistic federal poverty levels (FPLs) and draconian work requirements in non-expansion states. "Ample evidence exists, that work requirements don't achieve either of the goals their proponents hold dear: They don't reduce joblessness and they don't improve people's health. They reduce enrollment, in part because they typically come with administrative requirements that low-income households can't meet and the state bureaucracies can't handle."[30]

- Double the Marketplace open-enrollment period to ease the pressure on those who need adequate time to understand and choose the right plan.
- Reinstate the individual mandate to ease upward pressure on premiums for the entire pool of enrollees. Here's a fact that those on the right who oppose the ACA don't like to be reminded of: The personal mandate was originally promoted in the early 1990s by the Heritage Foundation, a conservative think tank.[31] As a knee-jerk reaction to "Hillarycare," it was conceived to prevent "a government takeover" of our insurance and promoted personal responsibility—unquestionably conservative pillars for their vision of America. The personal responsibility part was the individual mandate.

It was first sponsored and introduced on the floor of the U.S. Senate by Republican senator Don Nickles of Oklahoma (by no means a flaming liberal), plus twenty-four Republican cosponsors on November 20, 1993. The bill was named "Consumer Choice Health Security Act." On November 23, 1993, the bill's sponsor, Senator John Chafee (Republican from Rhode Island), introduced the Health Equity and Access Reform Today Act—cosponsored by eighteen of his Republican colleagues and two Democrats.

"If it will feed nothing else, it will feed my revenge."

—Shylock, *The Merchant of Venice* (1598)

I know what you're probably thinking about: that gleeful Rose Garden victory dance in May 2017 by Donald Trump and dozens of Republican lawmakers celebrating the repeal of the individual mandate they universally blamed on Obama. They either were ignorant or didn't care that the individual mandate not that long ago was birthed by Republicans and sacrosanct on their health insurance wish list.

Ironically, it took a Republican governor to first enshrine the individual mandate into law (albeit state law) as an integral part of what became Romneycare by the then Massachusetts governor, Mitt Romney, in 2006.

- Despite the increase in the number of those who now have health insurance since 2014, the number of those who are underinsured has increased to more than 97.8 million[32] due to higher deductibles and out-of-pocket maximums for plans through the Marketplace, private plans, and especially employer-provided ones. Since the government already subsidizes roughly $1.697 trillion per year to existing health insurance plans, why not convert a portion of those subsidies into a public option that could supplement those already with existing plans or those with no plan at all? It's time to help employees with the burden of too high deductibles and employees' portion of premiums.

- Reinstate funding for the Navigator and outreach programs that help in choosing and enrolling in the right Marketplace plan for the right individual.

- Ban short-term and association-based insurance plans that do not comply with the ten essential benefits of the ACA. Those plans mislead enrollees about their actual coverage, lead to higher premiums for those remaining in the Marketplace, and frequently collapse due to under-capitalization when enrollees need their benefits.

The Humiliation of Wanting to Live

For millions of people and their families, going through the nightmare of addiction, mental illness, or the battle with a potentially terminal disease such as cancer is difficult enough. And having to repeatedly prove medical necessity for life-saving treatment to an insurance company is an experience that millions of us have to bear. The constant struggle between medical professionals and a company whose very existence is based on the profit motive is an indignity piled on top of the terror, anguish, humiliation, and uncertainty that too many individuals and families are forced to endure. It is immoral. It is un-American. We can do better.

My friend Carole, who is the clinical director at a highly reputable rehab, struggles with insurance companies on a daily basis to continue medically necessary care for her patients. Little did she know that she would have to do the same for her own husband's life when he was struck with cancer. "Despite my expertise in working with insurance companies, it helped little when it came to fighting for a single case agreement when we discovered there were no in-network facilities specializing in his type of cancer. Navigating through the miasma of managed care networks added stress and valuable time that no family should have to endure when faced with true life or death decisions."[33]

According to the Americans with Disabilities Act (ADA) of 1990 and amended in 2008, addiction, mental illness, and terminal diseases are disabilities since they are "a physical or mental impairment that substantially limits one or more major life activities of such individual," and thus discriminatory. Furthermore, "Many people with physical or mental disabilities have been precluded from doing so because of discrimination." "Discrimination against individuals with disabilities persists in such critical areas as . . . health services."[34]

An insurance company's refusal to continue authorizing treatment considered medically necessary by an individual's attending health care professionals is discriminatory by definition since an insurance company is denying an individual life-saving treatment based on the treatment's cost. Plus, it violates our Constitution's Fourteenth Amendment, which guarantees "That no state [an insurance company must be licensed by the state in which it does business] shall . . . deprive any person of life, liberty or property, without due process of law."[35]

Seriously, if you are fighting a terminal disease and deprived of a particular treatment advocated by the doctors who are treating you because your insurance company says "no," who are you going to believe—your doctors or a company that is trying to cut costs?

As I described in chapter 5, through my clients, I have seen this issue way too many times, but there is a way to deal with it: establish treatment coverage for behavioral health and terminal diseases through a stand-alone program, a public plan, or Medicare. Treatment for life-threatening diseases for Americans of all ages should be considered a service, not a business. It is also an investment, an economic stimulus since only healthy citizens can grow a nation's economy.

And Finally

It doesn't take a genius to know that the best tool in helping those with SUDs and mental disorders is treatment. It also doesn't take a genius to recognize the myriad of studies proving that treatment provides net benefits way beyond its costs—and provides stimulus for economic growth. Want a healthy economy? Get people healthy.

If there is one thought with which I would like to wrap up this book, it is this: For those who are hit by addiction and/or mental illness, you are not alone—there is a treatment plan for you, no matter your socioeconomic situation. Only by recognizing there are others out there just like you and your family will you get through this ordeal.

Although we still have a long way to go, reach out for help; it is there for those who want and need it.

NOTES

Introduction

1. "Drugs at Work," National Safety Council, accessed January 2021, https://www.nsc.org/work-safety/safety-topics/drugs-at-work.

2. "Facing Addiction in America: The Surgeon General's Report on Alcohol, Drugs and Health," Office of the Surgeon General, November 2016, 2-2, https://store.samhsa.gov/product/Facing-Addiction-in-America-The-Surgeon-General-s-Report-on-Alcohol-Drugs-and-Health-Full-Report/SMA16-4991.

3. John LaRosa, "$42 Billion U.S. Addiction Rehab Industry Poised for Growth, and Challenges," Market Research.com, February 5, 2020, accessed March 1, 2020, https://blog.marketresearch.com/42-billion-u.s.-addiction-rehab-industry-poised-for-growth-and-challenges.

4. Debra Jay, *It Takes a Family: A Cooperative Approach to Lasting Sobriety* (Center City, MN: Hazelden, 2014), 9.

Chapter 1: Breaking the Glass

1. "Overdose Deaths Accelerating during COVID-19," Centers for Disease Control and Prevention, December 17, 2020, https://www.cdc.gov/media/releases/2020/p1218-overdose-deaths-covid-19.html.

2. "Facing Addiction in America: The Surgeon General's Report on Alcohol, Drugs and Health," Office of the Surgeon General, November

2016, 2-2, https://store.samhsa.gov/product/Facing-Addiction-in-America-The-Surgeon-General-s-Report-on-Alcohol-Drugs-and-Health-Full-Report/SMA16-4991.

Chapter 2: What Is Treatment?

1. "What Is Substance Abuse Treatment? A Booklet for Families," Substance Abuse and Mental Health Services Administration, January 2014, 3, https://store.samhsa.gov/product/What-Is-Substance-Abuse-Treatment-A-Booklet-for-Families/SMA14-4126.

2. "An Overview of Treatment Improvement Protocol (TIP) 63: Medications for Opioid Use Disorder," Substance Abuse and Mental Health Services Administration, February 1, 2018, ES-1, https://www.samhsa.gov/sites/default/files/programs_campaigns/kap/tip-63_overview_of_treatment_ppt_7-11-18.pptx.

3. Dr. Kevin McCauley, "The Brain and Recovery: An Update on the Neuroscience of Addiction," YouTube, May 4, 2018, https://www.youtube.com /watch?v=zYphZvRHm6Y.

4. "Facing Addiction in America: The Surgeon General's Report on Alcohol, Drugs and Health," Office of the Surgeon General, November 2016, 1, https://store.samhsa.gov/product/Facing-Addiction-in-America-The-Surgeon-General-s-Report-on-Alcohol-Drugs-and-Health-Full-Report/SMA16-4991.

5. "Opioid Overdose: Opioid Dispensing Rate Maps," Centers for Disease Control and Prevention, December 7, 2020, https://www.cdc.gov/drugoverdose/maps/rxrate-maps.html.

6. Elton John, "Elton John Recalls Performing for the First Time since Getting Sober: 'I Was Terrified,'" *Variety*, November 5, 2019, https://variety.com/2019/music/uncategorized/elton-john-sober-addiction-recovery-1203392566/.

7. "Drugs, Brains and Behavior: The Science of Addiction," National Institute on Drug Abuse, revised July 2018, https://www.drugabuse.gov/publications/drugs-brains-behavior-science-addiction/treatment-recovery.

8. Office of the Surgeon General, "Facing Addiction in America," 5-7.

9. William Cope Moyers, *Now What? An Insider's Guide to Addiction and Recovery* (Center City, MN: Hazelden, 2012), 83.

10. "Inspirational Quotes about Alcoholism," A Forever Recovery, https://aforeverrecovery.com/blog/information/inspirational-quotes-about-alcoholism/.

11. "Mental Illness," National Institute of Mental Health, https://www.nimh.nih.gov/health/statistics/mental-illness.shtml.

12. Debra Jay, *It Takes a Family: A Cooperative Approach to Lasting Sobriety* (Center City, MN: Hazelden, 2014), 8–9.

13. Linda A. Dimef and Marsha M. Linehan, "Dialectical Behavior Therapy for Substance Abusers," *Addiction Science and Clinical Practice* 4, no. 2 (June 2008): 39–47, https://www.ncbi.nlm.nih.gov/pmc/articles/PMC2797106/#.

14. "Dialectical Behavior Therapy (DBT)," Good Therapy, last updated June 13, 2018, https://www.goodtherapy.org/learn-about-therapy/types/dialectical-behavioral-therapy.

15. "What Are the Benefits of DBT?" Sierra Tucson, https://www.sierratucson.com/therapies/evidence-based/dialectical-behavioral/.

Chapter 3: The Right Rehab

1. "Rob Lowe Quotes," BrainyQuote, https://www.brainyquote.com/quotes/rob_lowe_177434.

2. "N-SSATS Facilities, by Status, Response Rate, Mode of Response, and State or Jurisdiction," table 6.1 in "National Survey of Substance Abuse Treatment Services (N-SSATS): 2019 Data on Substance Abuse Treatment Facilities," Substance Abuse and Mental Health Services Administration, August 20, 2020, https://www.samhsa.gov/data/sites/default/files/reports/rpt29389/2019_NSSATS/2019_NSSATS_Tables.html#Tbl6.1.

Chapter 4: Intervention

1. "J. K. Rowling > Quotes > Quotable Quotes," Goodreads, accessed May 25, 2021, https://www.goodreads.com/quotes/396385-rock-bottom-became-the-solid-foundation-on-which-i-rebuilt.

2. "What Is CRAFT?" Sober Families, 2019, https://www.soberfamilies.com/about-craft.

3. Shelly Lewis, "Addiction Is a Family Disease: One Person May Use, but the Whole Family Suffers," Alcohol Sayings, Liquor Quotes, accessed

May 25, 2021, http://www.alcoholsayings.com/addiction-is-a-family-dis ease-one-person-may-use-but-the-whole-family-suffers/.

4. Debra Jay, *It Takes a Family: A Cooperative Approach to Lasting Sobriety* (Center City, MN: Hazelden, 2014), 121.

5. Kendra Cherry, "The 6 Stages of Behavior Change: The Transtheoretical or Stages of Change Model," reviewed by Amy Morin, *Verywell Mind*, last updated November 19, 2020, https://www.verywellmind.com/the-stages-of-change-2794868.

6. Health Chitwood, personal communication with the author, January 24, 2021.

7. "5 Ways to Stop Enabling Your Loved One's Addiction," Circle of Hope, accessed May 25, 2021, https://circleofhopetreatment.com/2020/06/21/5-ways-to-stop-enabling-your-loved-ones-addiction/.

8. Jeffrey Klein, personal communication with the author, January 22, 2021.

Chapter 5: The Right Plan

1. "What Is Drug Addiction Treatment?" National Institute on Drug Abuse, September 18, 2020, https://www.drugabuse.gov/publications/principles-drug-addiction-treatment-research-based-guide-third-edition/frequently-asked-questions/what-drug-addiction-treatment.

2. Maria Shriver, *I've Been Thinking: Reflections, Prayers and Meditations for a Meaningful Life* (New York: Viking, 2018), 6.

3. "Facing Addiction in America: The Surgeon General's Report on Alcohol, Drugs and Health," Office of the Surgeon General, November 2016, 4-2, https://store.samhsa.gov/product/Facing-Addiction-in-America-The-Surgeon-General-s-Report-on-Alcohol-Drugs-and-Health-Full-Report/SMA16-4991.

4. "Seeking Drug Abuse Treatment: Know What to Ask," National Institute on Drug Abuse, June 2013, 5, https://www.drugabuse.gov/sites/default/files/treatmentbrochure_web.pdf.

5. "Medications for Opioid Use Disorder: For Healthcare and Addiction Professionals, Policymakers, Patients, and Families," Treatment Improvement Protocol (TIP) Series 63, Substance Abuse and Mental Health Services Administration, last updated 2020, ES-1, https://store.samhsa

.gov/product/TIP-63-Medications-for-Opioid-Use-Disorder-Full-Docu
ment/PEP20-02-01-006.

6. William Cope Moyers, *Now What? An Insider's Guide to Addiction
and Recovery* (Center City, MN: Hazelden, 2012), 82.

7. Rachel Miller, personal communication with the author, January
22, 2021.

8. Sara R. Collins, Munira Z. Gunja, and Gabriella N. Aboulafia, "U.S. Health Insurance Coverage in 2020: A Looming Crisis in
Affordability," Commonwealth Fund, August 19, 2020, https://www
.commonwealthfund.org/publications/issue-briefs/2020/aug/looming-cri
sis-health-coverage-2020-biennial.

9. "Detoxification and Substance Abuse Treatment," Treatment Improvement Protocol (TIP) Series 45, Substance Abuse and Mental Health
Services Administration, 2006, rev. 2015, https://store.samhsa.gov/system/
files/sma15-4131.pdf.

10. Office of the Surgeon General, "Facing Addiction in America,"
4-13.

11. "Types of Treatment Programs," National Institute on Drug Abuse,
January 2018, https://www.drugabuse.gov/publications/principles-drug
-addiction-treatment-research-based-guide-third-edition/drug-addiction
-treatment-in-united-states/types-treatment-programs.

12. Noam N. Levy, "Health Insurance Deductibles Soar, Leaving
Americans with Unaffordable Bills," *Los Angeles Times*, May 2, 2019,
https://www.latimes.com/politics/la-na-pol-health-insurance-medical
-bills-20190502-story.html.

13. Office of the Surgeon General, "Facing Addiction in America,"
4-31.

14. Office of the Surgeon General, "Facing Addiction in America," 5-11.

15. Michael Botticelli, "Remarks by ONDCP Director Michael Botticelli," White House, September 17, 2015, https://obamawhitehouse
.archives.gov/the-press-office/2015/09/17/remarks-ondcp-director-michael
-botticelli.

16. Office of the Surgeon General, "Facing Addiction in America,"
4-21.

17. "National Survey of Substance Abuse Treatment Services (N-
SSATS): 2019 Data on Substance Abuse Treatment Services," Sub-

stance Abuse and Mental Health Services Administration, August 20, 2020, table 2.4, https://www.samhsa.gov/data/sites/default/files/reports/rpt29389/2019_NSSATS/2019_NSSATS_Tables.html#TBl2.4.

18. Office of the Surgeon General, "Facing Addiction in America," 4-21.

19. Substance Abuse and Mental Health Services Administration, "Medications for Opioid Use Disorder," 1-8.

20. Office of the Surgeon General, "Facing Addiction in America," 4-21.

21. "What Science Tells Us about Opioid Use and Addiction," National Institute on Drug Abuse, January 27, 2016, https://www.drugabuse.gov/about-nida/legislative-activities/testimony-to-congress/2016/what-science-tells-us-about-opioid-abuse-and-addiction.

22. Pew Charitable Trusts, "Medication-Assisted Treatment Improves Outcomes for Patients with Opioid Use Disorder."

23. Office of the Surgeon General, "Facing Addiction in America," 4-24.

24. National Institute on Drug Abuse, "What Science Tells Us about Opioid Use and Addiction."

25. "Is the Use of Medications Like Methadone and Buprenorphine Simply Replacing One Addiction with Another?" National Institute on Drug Abuse, revised January 2018, https://www.drugabuse.gov/publications/principles-drug-addiction-treatment-research-based-guide-third-edition/frequently-asked-questions/use-medications-methadone-buprenorphine.

26. German Lopez, "There's a Highly Successful Treatment for Opioid Addiction: But Stigma Is Holding It Back," *Vox*, November 15, 2017, https://www.vox.com/science-and-health/2017/7/20/15937896/medication-assisted-treatment-methadone-buprenorphine-naltrexone.

27. Lopez, "There's a Highly Successful Treatment for Opioid Addiction."

28. Office of the Surgeon General, "Facing Addiction in America," 4-22, 6-6.

29. We Are Not Saints, https://wearenotsaints.com/.

30. "Historical Data: The Birth of A.A. and Its Growth in the U.S./Canada," Alcoholics Anonymous, https://www.aa.org/pages/en_US/historical-data-the-birth-of-aa-and-its-growth-in-the-uscanada.

31. Office of the Surgeon General, "Facing Addiction in America," 5-9.

32. Office of the Surgeon General, "Facing Addiction in America," 5-9.

33. Debra Jay, *It Takes a Family: A Cooperative Approach to Lasting Sobriety* (Center City, MN: Hazelden, 2014), 122.

34. Office of the Surgeon General, "Facing Addiction in America," 5-10.

35. Office of the Surgeon General, "Facing Addiction in America," 2-2.

36. Karin Swenson, personal communication with the author, March 22, 2020.

Chapter 6: How to Get Treatment

1. "Mahatma Gandhi Quotes," Quotefancy, accessed May 25, 2021, https://quotefancy.com/mahatma-gandhi-quotes.

2. "Key Substance Use and Mental Health Indicators in the United States: Results from the 2019 National Survey on Drug Use and Health," Substance Abuse and Mental Health Services Administration, September 2020, 3-4, https://www.samhsa.gov/data/report/2019-nsduh-annual-national-report.

3. Ruixuan Jiang, Inyoung Lee, Todd A. Lee, and A. Simon Pickard, "The Societal Cost of Heroin Use Disorder in the United States," *PloS ONE*, May 30, 2017, https://journals.plos.org/plosone/article?id=10.1371/journal.pone.0177323.

4. Dylan Matthews, "Everything You Need to Know about the War on Poverty," *Washington Post*, January 8, 2014, https://www.washingtonpost.com/news/wonk/wp/2014/01/08/everything-you-need-to-know-about-the-war-on-poverty/.

5. Matthews, "War on Poverty."

6. Matthews, "War on Poverty."

7. Melissa Linebaugh, "SSDI and SSI Disability Benefit for Drug Addiction," Disability Secrets, accessed January 30, 2021, https://www.disabilitysecrets.com/social-security-disability-drug-addiction.html.

8. "Income Level and Savings," Healthcare.gov, https://www.healthcare.gov/lower-costs/.

9. Healthcare.gov, https://www.healthcare.gov/income-and-household-information/income/#magi.

10. "Facing Addiction in America: The Surgeon General's Report on Alcohol, Drugs and Health," Office of the Surgeon General, November 2016, 6-25, https://store.samhsa.gov/product/Facing-Addiction-in-Amer ica-The-Surgeon-General-s-Report-on-Alcohol-Drugs-and-Health-Full -Report/SMA16-4991.

11. "Medicaid and CHIP Eligibility, Enrollment and Cost-Sharing Policies as of January 2021," Kaiser Family Foundation, http://files.kff.org/ attachment/Table-4-Medicaid-and-CHIP-Eligibility-as-of-Jan-2020.pdf.

12. "What Is the Spending on Medicare?" US Government Spending, January 4, 2021, https://www.usgovernmentspending.com/medi care_spending_by_year#:~:text=In%20FY%202020%20the%20 federal,collections%2C%E2%80%9D%20was%20%24924%20billion.

13. Healthcare.gov, https://www.healthcare.gov/income-and-house hold-information/income/#magi.

14. Jennifer Tolbert and Kendal Orgera, "Key Facts about the Uninsured Population," Kaiser Family Foundation, December 7, 2018, https://www .kff.org/uninsured/fact-sheet/key-facts-about-the-uninsured-population/.

15. "4.7 Million Uninsured Adults Could Become Eligible for Medicaid by 2021 if All Remaining States Expanded the Program under the ACA," Kaiser Family Foundation, June 25, 2020, https://www.kff.org/uninsured/ press-release/4-7-million-uninsured-adults-could-become-eligible-for -medicaid-by-2021-if-all-remaining-states-expanded-the-program-under -the-aca/.

16. Robin Rudowitz, Rachel Garfield, and Elizabeth Hinton, "10 Things to Know about Medicaid: Setting the Facts Straight," Kaiser Family Foundation, March 6, 2019, https://www.kff.org/medicaid/issue -brief/10-things-to-know-about-medicaid-setting-the-facts-straight/.

17. Louise Norris, "Medicaid Coverage in Your State," Healthinsur ance.org, February 18, 2019, https://www.healthinsurance.org/medicaid/.

18. Sara R. Collins, Munira Z. Gunja, and Gabriella N. Aboula fia, "U.S. Health Insurance Coverage in 2020: A Looming Crisis in Affordability," Commonwealth Fund, August 19, 2020, https://www .commonwealthfund.org/publications/issue-briefs/2020/aug/looming-cri sis-health-coverage-2020-biennial.

19. Austin Frakt, "A Sense of Alarm as Rural Hospitals Keep Closing," *New York Times*, October 20, 2018, https://www.nytimes.com/2018/10/29/ upshot/a-sense-of-alarm-as-rural-hospitals-keep-closing.html.

20. "What's Medicare?" Medicare.gov, https://www.medicare.gov/what-medicare-covers/your-medicare-coverage-choices/whats-medicare.

21. "What Is Medicare: Essential Medicare Facts You Should Know," eHealth Medicare, https://www.ehealthmedicare.com/about-medicare-articles/facts-about-medicare/.

22. "Medicare-Covered Services: Mental Health Services," Medicare Interactive, https://www.medicareinteractive.org/get-answers/medicare-covered-services/mental-health-services.

23. Medicare Interactive, "Medicare-Covered Services."

24. Daniel L. Dickerson, Suzanne Spear, Pamela Marinelli-Casey, Richard Rawson, Libo Li, and Yih-Ing Hser, "American Indians / Alaska Natives and Substance Use Treatment Outcomes: Positive Signs and Continuing Challenges," NCBI, January 2011, https://www.ncbi.nlm.nih.gov/pmc/articles/PMC3042549/.

25. Wendy Sawyer and Peter Wagner, "Mass Incarceration: The Whole Pie 2019," Prison Policy Initiative, March 19, 2019, https://www.prisonpolicy.org/reports/pie2019.html.

26. "2018 Crime in the United States," Federal Bureau of Investigation, https://ucr.fbi.gov/crime-in-the-u.s/2018/crime-in-the-u.s.-2018/topic-pages/persons-arrested.

27. Matthes Friedman, "Just Facts: As Many Americans Have Criminal Records as College Diplomas," Brennan Center for Justice, November 17, 2015, https://www.brennancenter.org/blog/just-facts-many-americans-have-criminal-records-college-diplomas.

28. Office of the Surgeon General, "Facing Addiction in America," 6-19.

29. Kenneth Stoner, "Need to Know," KTLV AM Radio, March 2018.

30. Austin Frakt, "Spend a Dollar on Drug Treatment, and Save More on Crime Reduction," *New York Times*, April 24, 2017, https://www.nytimes.com/2017/04/24/upshot/spend-a-dollar-on-drug-treatment-and-save-more-on-crime-reduction.html?_r=0.

31. Hefi Wen, Jason M. Hockenberry, and Janet R. Cummings, "The Effect of Substance Use Disorder Treatment Use on Crime: Evidence from Public Insurance Expansions and Health Insurance Mandates," NBER Working Paper 20537, October 2014, abstract, https://www.nber.org/papers/w20537.pdf.

32. Frakt, "Spend a Dollar on Drug Treatment."

33. Samuel R. Bondurant, Jason M. Lindo, and Isaac D. Swensen, "Substance Abuse Treatment Centers and Local Crime," NBER Working Paper 22610, 4, September 2016, https://www.nber.org/papers/w22610.pdf.

34. Mena Samara, personal communication with the author, January 24, 2021.

35. Ed Blau, personal communication with the author, January 18, 2021.

Chapter 7: Cheat Sheet: A Summary of What You Need to Know Now-Now

1. Dr. Kevin McCauley, "The Brain and Recovery: An Update on the Neuroscience of Addiction," YouTube, May 4, 2018, https://www.you tube.com/watch?v=zYphZvRHm6Y.

2. "Drugs, Brains and Behavior: The Science of Addiction," National Institute on Drug Abuse, revised July 2018, https://www.drugabuse.gov/publications/drugs-brains-behavior-science-addiction/treatment-recovery.

3. "Facing Addiction in America: The Surgeon General's Report on Alcohol, Drugs and Health," Office of the Surgeon General, November 2016, 5-7, https://store.samhsa.gov/product/Facing-Addiction-in-America-The-Surgeon-General-s-Report-on-Alcohol-Drugs-and-Health-Full-Report/SMA16-4991.

4. "Mental Illness," National Institute of Mental Health, https://www.nimh.nih.gov/health/statistics/mental-illness.shtml.

5. Office of the Surgeon General, "Facing Addiction in America," 5-3.

6. "Is the Use of Medications Like Methadone and Buprenorphine Simply Replacing One Addiction with Another?" National Institute on Drug Abuse, revised January 2018, https://www.drugabuse.gov/publications/principles-drug-addiction-treatment-research-based-guide-third-edition/frequently-asked-questions/use-medications-methadone-buprenorphine-simply-replacing.

7. "National Survey of Substance Abuse Treatment Services (N-SSATS): 2019 Data on Substance Abuse Treatment Services," Substance Abuse and Mental Health Services Administration, August 20, 2020, table 2.4, https://www.samhsa.gov/data/sites/default/files/reports/rpt29389/2019_NSSATS/2019_NSSATS_Tables.html#Tbl2.4.

8. Office of the Surgeon General, "Facing Addiction in America," 5-9.

9. Office of the Surgeon General, "Facing Addiction in America," 4.

10. Office of the Surgeon General, "Facing Addiction in America," 2-2.

Chapter 8: Aftermath: What We Need to Do

1. "Key Substance Use and Mental Health Indicators in the United States: Results from the 2019 National Survey on Drug Use and Health," Substance Abuse and Mental Health Services Administration, September 2020, 50–52, https://www.samhsa.gov/data/report/2019-nsduh-annual -national-report.

2. Rachel Garfield, Kendal Orgera, and Anthony Damico, "The Uninsured and the ACA: A Primer—Key Facts about Health Insurance and the Uninsured amidst Changes to the Affordable Care Act," Kaiser Family Foundation, January 25, 2019, https://www.kff.org/uninsured/report/the -uninsured-and-the-aca-a-primer-key-facts-about-health-insurance-and -the-uninsured-amidst-changes-to-the-affordable-care-act/.

3. "Detoxification and Substance Abuse Treatment," Treatment Improvement Protocol (TIP) Series 45, P42, Substance Abuse and Mental Health Services Administration, 2006, revised 2015, https://store.samhsa .gov/system/files/sma15-4131.pdf.

4. "Teaching Addiction Science: Understanding Drug Abuse and Addiction: What Science Says," National Institute on Drug Abuse, February 2016, https://www.drugabuse.gov/publications/teaching-addiction -science/understanding-drug-abuse-addiction-what-science-says.

5. Susan L. Ettner, David Huang, Elizabeth Evans, Danielle Rose Ash, Mary Hardy, Mickel Jourabchi, and Yih-Ing Hser, "Benefit–Cost in the California Treatment Outcome Project: Does Substance Abuse Treatment 'Pay for Itself?'" Health Services Research 41, no. 1 (2006): 192–213, https://www.ncbi.nlm.nih.gov/pmc/articles/PMC1681530/.

6. Ettner et al., "Benefit–Cost in the California Treatment Outcome Project," abstract.

7. Nicole Lewis and Beatrix Lockwood, "The Hidden Cost of Incarceration," Marshall Project, December 17, 2019, https://www.themarshall project.org.

8. National Institute on Drug Abuse, "Teaching Addiction Science."

9. "Benefit-Cost Results," Washington State Institute for Public Policy, accessed May 26, 2021, http://www.wsipp.wa.gov/BenefitCost?topicId=7.

10. Washington State Institute for Public Policy, "Benefit-Cost Results."

11. For all results, see Washington State Institute for Public Policy, "Benefit-Cost Results."

12. Jennifer Tolbert, Kendal Orgera, and Anthony Damico, "Key Facts about the Uninsured Population," Kaiser Family Foundation, November 6, 2020, https://www.kff.org/uninsured/issue-brief/key-facts-about-the -uninsured-population/.

13. Phil Galewitz, "Breaking a Ten-Year Streak: The Number of Uninsured Americans Rises," Kaiser Health News, September 10, 2019, https:// khn.org/news/number-of-americans-without-insurance-rises-in-2018/.

14. "Federal Subsidies for Health Insurance Coverage for People under Age 65: 2019 to 2029," Congressional Budget Office, May 2019, https://www.cbo.gov/system/files/2019-05/55085-HealthCoverageSub sidies_0.pdf.

15. Lauren Weber, "How Political Maneuvering Derailed a Red State's Path to Medicaid Expansion," Kaiser Health News, September 6, 2019, https://khn.org/news/kansas-medicaid-expansion-conservative-political -playbook/.

16. Galewitz, "Breaking a Ten-Year Streak."

17. Sarah Miller, Norman Johnson, and Laura R. Wherry, "Medicaid and Mortality: New Evidence from Linked Survey and Administrative Data," National Bureau of Economic Research, revised January 2021, https://www.nber.org/papers/w26081.

18. Jessica Schubel and Matt Broaddus, "Uncompensated Care Costs Fell in Nearly Every State as ACA's Major Coverage Provisions Took Effect," Center on Budget and Policy Priorities, May 23, 2018, https://www .cbpp.org/research/health/uncompensated-care-costs-fell-in-nearly-every -state-as-acas-major-coverage.

19. Julia Zur, MaryBeth Musumeci, and Rachel Garfield, "Medicaid's Role in Financing Behavioral Health Services for Low-Income Individuals," Kaiser Family Foundation, June 29, 2017, https://www.kff. org/report-section/medicaids-role-in-financing-behavioral-health-services -for-low-income-individuals-issue-brief/.

20. Tolbert, Orgera, and Damico, "Key Facts about the Uninsured Population."

21. Luojia Hu, Robert Kaestner, Bhashkar Mazumder, Sarah Miller, and Ashley Wong, "The Effect of the Affordable Care Act Medicaid Expan-

sions on Financial Wellbeing," *Journal of Public Economics* 163 (July 2018): 99–112, https://www.ncbi.nlm.nih.gov/pmc/articles/PMC6208351/.

22. Institute of Medicine (US) Committee on the Consequences of Uninsurance, *Hidden Costs, Values Lost: Uninsurance in America* (Washington, DC: National Academies Press, 2003), https://www.ncbi.nlm.nih.gov/books/NBK221662/.

23. Hu et al., "The Effect of the Affordable Care Act Medicaid Expansions on Financial Wellbeing."

24. Stanley F. Hupfeld, *Political Malpractice: How the Politicians Made a Mess of Health Reform* (Tulsa, OK: Yorkshire, 2018), 24.

25. Daniel Rivero, "Why Calling Obamacare 'Socialism' Makes No Sense [Analysis]," ABC News, October 1, 2013, https://abcnews.go.com/ABC_Univision/Politics/calling-obamacare-socialism-makes-sense-analysis/story?id=20435162.

26. Ayla Ellison, "16 Rural Hospital Closures in 2020," Becker's Hospital Review, October 29, 2020, https://www.beckershospitalreview.com/finance/16-rural-hospital-closures-in-2020.html.

27. "176 Rural Hospital Closures: January 2005–Present (134 since 2010)," Cecil G. Sheps Center for Health Services Research, https://www.shepscenter.unc.edu/programs-projects/rural-health/rural-hospital-closures/.

28. Austin Frakt, "A Sense of Alarm as Rural Hospitals Keep Closing," *New York Times*, October 20, 2018, https://www.nytimes.com/2018/10/29/upshot/a-sense-of-alarm-as-rural-hospitals-keep-closing.html.

29. Sara Barry, personal communication with the author, January 14, 2021.

30. Michel Hiltzik,"Trump Launches Sneaky 11th-Hour Attacks on Clean Air, Medicaid and LGBTQ People," *Los Angeles Times*, January 14, 2020, https://www.latimes.com/business/story/2021-01-14/trump-sneaky-attacks-clean-air-medicaid-lgbtq.

31. Avik Roy and The Apothecary, "How the Heritage Foundation, a Conservative Think Tank, Promoted the Individual Mandate," *Forbes*, October 20, 2011, https://www.forbes.com/sites/theapothecary/2011/10/20/how-a-conservative-think-tank-invented-the-individual-mandate/#6e49786c6187.

32. Hu et al., "The Effect of the Affordable Care Act Medicaid Expansions on Financial Wellbeing."

33. Anonymous, personal communication with the author, January 24, 2021.

34. "Americans with Disabilities Act of 1990 as Amended," https://www.ada.gov/pubs/adastatute08.htm#12101a.

35. "U.S. Constitution > 14th Amendment," Legal Information Institute, https://www.law.cornell.edu/constitution/amendmentxiv.

BIBLIOGRAPHY

Alcoholics Anonymous. "Historical Data: The Birth of A.A. and Its Growth in the U.S./Canada." https://www.aa.org/pages/en_US/histori cal-data-the-birth-of-aa-and-its-growth-in-the-uscanada.

"Americans with Disabilities Act of 1990 as Amended." https://www.ada .gov/pubs/adastatute08.htm#12101a.

Bondurant, Samuel R., Jason M. Lindo, and Isaac D. Swensen. "Substance Abuse Treatment Centers and Local Crime." NBER Working Paper 22610. September 2016. https://www.nber.org/papers/w22610.pdf.

Botticelli, Michael. "Remarks by ONDCP Director Michael Botticelli." White House, September 17, 2015. https://obamawhitehouse.archives .gov/the-press-office/2015/09/17/remarks-ondcp-director-michael-bot ticelli.

BrainyQuote. "Rob Lowe Quotes." https://www.brainyquote.com/quotes/ rob_lowe_177434.

Broaddus, Matt, and Aviva Aron-Dine. "Medicaid Expansion Has Saved at Least 19,200 Lives, New Research Finds." Center on Budget and Policy Priorities, November 6, 2019. https://www.cbpp.org/research/health/ medicaid-expansion-has-saved-at-least-19000-lives-new-research-finds.

Cecil G. Sheps Center for Health Services Research. "176 Rural Hospital Closures: January 2005–Present (134 since 2010)." https://www.sheps center.unc.edu/programs-projects/rural-health/rural-hospital-closures/.

Center for Behavioral Health Statistics and Quality. "Results from the 2019 National Survey on Drug Use and Health: Detailed Tables." 2020.

Table 5.28A: https://www.samhsa.gov/data/sites/default/files/reports/
rpt29394/NSDUHDetailedTabs2019/NSDUHDetTabsSect5pe2019.
htm#tab5-28a. Table 5.28B: https://www.samhsa.gov/data/sites/de
fault/files/reports/rpt29394/NSDUHDetailedTabs2019/NSDUHDet
TabsSect5pe2019.htm#tab5-28b.

Centers for Disease Control and Prevention. "Opioid Overdose: Opioid
Dispensing Rate Maps." December 7, 2020. https://www.cdc.gov/
drugoverdose/maps/rxrate-maps.html.

———. "Overdose Deaths Accelerating during COVID-19." December
17, 2020. https://www.cdc.gov/media/releases/2020/p1218-overdose
-deaths-covid-19.html.

Cherry, Kendra. "The 6 Stages of Behavior Change: The Transtheoretical
or Stages of Change Model." Reviewed by Amy Morin. *Verywell Mind*,
last updated November 19, 2020. https://www.verywellmind.com/the
-stages-of-change-2794868.

Circle of Hope. "5 Ways to Stop Enabling Your Loved One's Addiction." Accessed May 25, 2021. https://circleofhopetreatment
.com/2020/06/21/5-ways-to-stop-enabling-your-loved-ones-addiction/.

Collins, Sara R., Munira Z. Gunja, and Gabriella N. Aboulafia. "U.S.
Health Insurance Coverage in 2020: A Looming Crisis in Affordability."
Commonwealth Fund, August 19, 2020. https://www.commonwealth
fund.org/publications/issue-briefs/2020/aug/looming-crisis-health-cov
erage-2020-biennial.

Congress of the United States Congressional Budget Office. "Federal
Subsidies for Health Insurance Coverage for People under Age 65: 2019
to 2029." May 2019. https://www.cbo.gov/system/files/2019-05/55085
-HealthCoverageSubsidies_0.pdf.

Dickerson, Daniel L., Suzanne Spear, Pamela Marinelli-Casey, Richard
Rawson, Libo Li, and Yih-Ing Hser. "American Indians / Alaska Natives and Substance Use Treatment Outcomes: Positive Signs and Continuing Challenges." NCBI, January 2011. https://www.ncbi.nlm.nih
.gov/pmc/articles/PMC3042549/.

Dimef, Linda A., and Marsha M. Linehan. "Dialectical Behavior Therapy for Substance Abusers." *Addiction Science and Clinical Practice* 4,
no. 2 (June 2008): 39–47. https://www.ncbi.nlm.nih.gov/pmc/articles/
PMC2797106/#.

eHealth Medicare. "What Is Medicare: Essential Medicare Facts You Should Know." https://www.ehealthmedicare.com/about-medicare-articles/facts-about-medicare/.

Ellison, Ayla. "16 Rural Hospital Closures in 2020." Becker's Hospital Review, October 29, 2020. https://www.beckershospitalreview.com/finance/16-rural-hospital-closures-in-2020.html.

Ettner, Susan L., David Huang, Elizabeth Evans, Danielle Rose Ash, Mary Hardy, Mickel Jourabchi, and Yih-Ing Hser. "Benefit–Cost in the California Treatment Outcome Project: Does Substance Abuse Treatment 'Pay for Itself'?" *Health Services Research* 41, no. 1 (2006): 192–213. https://www.ncbi.nlm.nih.gov/pmc/articles/PMC1681530/.

Federal Bureau of Investigation. "2018 Crime in the United States." https://ucr.fbi.gov/crime-in-the-u.s/2018/crime-in-the-u.s.-2018/topic-pages/persons-arrested.

A Forever Recovery. "Inspirational Quotes about Alcoholism." https://aforeverrecovery.com/blog/information/ inspirational-quotes-about-alcoholism/.

Frakt, Austin. "A Sense of Alarm as Rural Hospitals Keep Closing." *New York Times*, October 20, 2018. https://www.nytimes.com/2018/10/29/upshot/a-sense-of-alarm-as-rural-hospitals-keep-closing.html.

———. "Spend a Dollar on Drug Treatment, and Save More on Crime Reduction." *New York Times*, April 24, 2017. https://www.nytimes.com/2017/04/24/upshot/spend-a-dollar-on-drug-treatment-and-save-more-on-crime-reduction.html?_r=0.

Friedman, Matthes. "Just Facts: As Many Americans Have Criminal Records as College Diplomas." Brennan Center for Justice, November 17, 2015. https://www.brennancenter.org/blog/just-facts-many-americans-have-criminal-records-college-diplomas.

Galewitz, Phil. "Breaking a Ten-Year Streak: The Number of Uninsured Americans Rises." Kaiser Health News, September 10, 2019. https://khn.org/news/number-of-americans-without-insurance-rises-in-2018/.

Garfield, Rachel, Kendal Orgera, and Anthony Damico. "The Uninsured and the ACA: A Primer—Key Facts about Health Insurance and the Uninsured amidst Changes to the Affordable Care Act." Kaiser Family Foundation, January 25, 2019. https://www.kff.org/uninsured/report/the-uninsured-and-the-aca-a-primer-key-facts-about-health-insurance-and-the-uninsured-amidst-changes-to-the-affordable-care-act/.

Garfield, Rachel, Robin Rudowitz, and Anthony Damico. "How Many Uninsured Adults Could Be Reached if All States Expanded Medicaid?" Kaiser Family Foundation, June 25, 2020. https://www.kff.org/report -section/how-many-uninsured-adults-could-be-reached-if-all-states-ex panded-medicaid-tables/.

Good Therapy. "Dialectical Behavior Therapy (DBT)." Last updated June 13, 2018. https://www.goodtherapy.org/learn-about-therapy/types/ dialectical-behavioral-therapy.

Goodreads. "J. K. Rowling > Quotes > Quotable Quotes." Accessed May 25, 2021. https://www.goodreads.com/quotes/396385-rock-bottom -became-the-solid-foundation-on-which-i-rebuilt.

Healthcare.gov. "Income Level and Savings." https://www.healthcare.gov/ lower-costs/.

Hiltzik, Michel. "Trump Launches Sneaky 11th-Hour Attacks on Clean Air, Medicaid and LGBTQ People." *Los Angeles Times*, January 14, 2020. https://www.latimes.com/business/story/2021-01-14/trump -sneaky-attacks-clean-air-medicaid-lgbtq.

Hu, Luojia, Robert Kaestner, Bhashkar Mazumder, Sarah Miller, and Ashley Wong. "The Effect of the Affordable Care Act Medicaid Expansions on Financial Wellbeing." *Journal of Public Economics* 163 (July 2018): 99–112. https://www.ncbi.nlm.nih.gov/pmc/articles/PMC6208351/.

Hupfeld, Stanley F. *Political Malpractice: How the Politicians Made a Mess of Health Reform*. Tulsa, OK: Yorkshire, 2018.

Institute of Medicine (US) Committee on the Consequences of Uninsurance. *Hidden Costs, Values Lost: Uninsurance in America*. Washington, DC: National Academies Press, 2003. https://www.ncbi.nlm.nih.gov/ books/NBK221662/.

Jay, Debra. *It Takes a Family: A Cooperative Approach to Lasting Sobriety*. Center City, MN: Hazelden, 2014.

Jiang, Ruixuan, Inyoung Lee, Todd A. Lee, and A. Simon Pickard. "The Societal Cost of Heroin Use Disorder in the United States." *PloS ONE*, May 30, 2017. https://journals.plos.org/plosone/article?id=10.1371/ journal.pone.0177323.

John, Elton. "Elton John Recalls Performing for the First Time since Getting Sober: 'I Was Terrified.'" *Variety*, November 5, 2019. https:// variety.com/2019/music/uncategorized/elton-john-sober-addiction-re covery-1203392566/.

Kaiser Family Foundation. "4.7 Million Uninsured Adults Could Become Eligible for Medicaid by 2021 if All Remaining States Expanded the Program under the ACA." KFF.org, June 25, 2020. https://www.kff .org/uninsured/press-release/4-7-million-uninsured-adults-could-be come-eligible-for-medicaid-by-2021-if-all-remaining-states-expanded -the-program-under-the-aca.

———. "Medicaid and CHIP Eligibility, Enrollment and Cost-Sharing Policies as of January 2021." KFF.org, http://files.kff.org/attachment/ Table-4-Medicaid-and-CHIP-Eligibility-as-of-Jan-2020.pdf.

Kentucky Health Benefit Exchange. "2021 Federal Poverty Level Chart." Last updated August 8, 2020. https://healthbenefitexchange.ky.gov/ About/Documents/2021-Federal-Poverty-Level-Chart.pdf.

LaRosa, John. "$42 Billion U.S. Addiction Rehab Industry Poised for Growth, and Challenges." Market Research.com, February 5, 2020. Accessed March 1, 2020. https://blog.marketresearch.com/42-billion-u.s. -addiction-rehab-industry-poised-for-growth-and-challenges.

Lawford, Christopher Kennedy. *Recover to Live: Kick Any Habit, Manage Any Addiction*. Dallas, TX: BenBella Books, 2013.

Legal Information Institute. "U.S. Constitution > 14th Amendment." https://www.law.cornell.edu/constitution/amendmentxiv.

Levy, Noam N. "Health Insurance Deductibles Soar, Leaving Americans with Unaffordable Bills." *Los Angeles Times*, May 2, 2019. https:// www.latimes.com/politics/la-na-pol-health-insurance-medical-bills -20190502-story.html.

Lewis, Nicole, and Beatrix Lockwood. "The Hidden Cost of Incarceration." Marshall Project, December 17, 2019. https://www.themarshall project.org.

Lewis, Shelly. "Addiction Is a Family Disease: One Person May Use, but the Whole Family Suffers." Alcohol Sayings, Liquor Quotes, accessed May 25, 2021. http://www.alcoholsayings.com/addiction-is-a-family -disease-one-person-may-use-but-the-whole-family-suffers/.

Linebaugh, Melissa. "SSDI and SSI Disability Benefit for Drug Addiction." Disability Secrets, accessed January 30, 2021. https://www.dis abilitysecrets.com/social-security-disability-drug-addiction.html.

Lopez, German. "There's a Highly Successful Treatment for Opioid Addiction: But Stigma Is Holding It Back." *Vox*, November 15, 2017.

https://www.vox.com/science-and-health/2017/7/20/15937896/medi
cation-assisted-treatment-methadone-buprenorphine-naltrexone.

Matthews, Dylan. "Everything You Need to Know about the War on Poverty." *Washington Post*, January 8, 2014. https://www.washingtonpost
.com/news/wonk/wp/2014/01/08/everything-you-need-to-know-about
-the-war-on-poverty/.

McCauley, Kevin. "The Brain and Recovery: An Update on the Neuroscience of Addiction." YouTube, May 4, 2018. https://www.youtube.com/
watch?v=zYphZvRHm6Y.

Medicare.gov. "What's Medicare?" https://www.medicare.gov/what-medi
care-covers/your-medicare-coverage-choices/whats-medicare.

Medicare Interactive. "Medicare-Covered Services: Mental Health Services." https://www.medicareinteractive.org/get-answers/medicare-cov
ered-services/mental-health-services.

Miller, Sarah, Norman Johnson, and Laura R. Wherry. "Medicaid and Mortality: New Evidence from Linked Survey and Administrative Data." National Bureau of Economic Research, revised January 2021. https://www.nber.org/papers/w26081.

Moyers, William Cope. *Now What? An Insider's Guide to Addiction and Recovery.* Center City, MN: Hazelden, 2012.

National Institute of Mental Health. "Mental Illness." https://www.nimh
.nih.gov/health/statistics/mental-illness.shtml.

National Institute on Drug Abuse. "Drugs, Brains and Behavior: The Science of Addiction." Revised July 2018. https://www.drugabuse.gov/pub
lications/drugs-brains-behavior-science-addiction/treatment-recovery.

———. "How Effective Is Drug Abuse Treatment?" Revised January 2018. https://www.drugabuse.gov/publications/principles-drug-addic
tion-treatment-research-based-guide-third-edition/frequently-asked
-questions/how-effective-drug-addiction-treatment.

———. "Is the Use of Medications Like Methadone and Buprenorphine Simply Replacing One Addiction with Another?" Revised January 2018. https://www.drugabuse.gov/publications/principles-drug-addiction
-treatment-research-based-guide-third-edition/frequently-asked-ques
tions/use-medications-methadone-buprenorphine-simply-replacing.

———. "Seeking Drug Abuse Treatment: Know What to Ask." June 2013. https://www.drugabuse.gov/sites/default/files/treatmentbrochure_web.pdf.

———. "Teaching Addiction Science: Understanding Drug Abuse and Addiction: What Science Says." February 2016. https://www.drug abuse.gov/publications/teaching-addiction-science/understanding-drug -abuse-addiction-what-science-says.

———. "Types of Treatment Programs." January 2018. https://www.dru-gabuse.gov/publications/principles-drug-addiction-treatment-research -based-guide-third-edition/drug-addiction-treatment-in-united-states/ types-treatment-programs.

———. "What Is Drug Addiction Treatment?" September 18, 2020. https://www.drugabuse.gov/publications/principles-drug-addiction -treatment-research-based-guide-third-edition/frequently-asked-ques tions/what-drug-addiction-treatment.

———. "What Science Tells Us about Opioid Use and Addiction." January 27, 2016. https://www.drugabuse.gov/about-nida/legislative-activities/ testimony-to-congress/2016/what-science-tells-us-about-opioid-abuse -and-addiction.

National Safety Council. "Drugs at Work." Accessed January 2021. https:// www.nsc.org/work-safety/safety-topics/drugs-at-work.

Norris, Louise. "Medicaid Coverage in Your State." Healthinsurance.org, February 18, 2019. https://www.healthinsurance.org/medicaid/.

Office of the Surgeon General. "Facing Addiction in America: The Surgeon General's Report on Alcohol, Drugs and Health." November 2016. https://store.samhsa.gov/product/Facing-Addiction-in-America -The-Surgeon-General-s-Report-on-Alcohol-Drugs-and-Health-Full -Report/SMA16-4991.

Pew Charitable Trusts. "Medication-Assisted Treatment Improves Outcomes for Patients with Opioid Use Disorder." November 22, 2016. https://www.pewtrusts.org/en/research-and-analysis/fact -sheets/2016/11/medication-assisted-treatment-improves-outcomes-for -patients-with-opioid-use-disorder.

Quotefancy. "Mahatma Gandhi Quotes." Accessed May 25, 2021. https:// quotefancy.com/mahatma-gandhi-quotes.

Rivero, Daniel. "Why Calling Obamacare 'Socialism' Makes No Sense [Analysis]." ABC News, October 1, 2013. https://abcnews.go.com/ ABC_Univision/Politics/calling-obamacare-socialism-makes-sense -analysis/story?id=20435162.

Roy, Avik, and The Apothecary. "How the Heritage Foundation, a Conservative Think Tank, Promoted the Individual Mandate." *Forbes*, October 20, 2011. https://www.forbes.com/sites/theapothe cary/2011/10/20/how-a-conservative-think-tank-invented-the-individ ual-mandate/#6e49786c6187.

Rudowitz, Robin, Rachel Garfield, and Elizabeth Hinton. "10 Things to Know about Medicaid: Setting the Facts Straight." Kaiser Family Foundation, March 6, 2019. https://www.kff.org/medicaid/issue-brief/10 -things-to-know-about-medicaid-setting-the-facts-straight/.

Sawyer, Wendy, and Peter Wagner. "Mass Incarceration: The Whole Pie 2019." Prison Policy Initiative, March 19, 2019. https://www.prison policy.org/reports/pie2019.html.

Schubel, Jessica, and Matt Broaddus. "Uncompensated Care Costs Fell in Nearly Every State as ACA's Major Coverage Provisions Took Effect." Center on Budget and Policy Priorities, May 23, 2018. https://www .cbpp.org/research/health/uncompensated-care-costs-fell-in-nearly-ev ery-state-as-acas-major-coverage.

Shriver, Maria. *I've Been Thinking: Reflections, Prayers and Meditations for a Meaningful Life*. New York: Viking, 2018.

Sierra Tucson. "What Are the Benefits of DBT?" https://www.sierratuc son.com/therapies/evidence-based/dialectical-behavioral/.

Sober Families. "What Is CRAFT?" 2019. https://www.soberfamilies .com/about-craft.

Stoner, Kenneth. "Need to Know." KTLV AM Radio, March 2018.

Substance Abuse and Mental Health Services Administration. "Detoxification and Substance Abuse Treatment." Treatment Improvement Protocol (TIP) Series 45. 2006. Revised 2015. https://store.samhsa.gov/ system/files/sma15-4131.pdf.

———. "Key Substance Use and Mental Health Indicators in the United States: Results from the 2019 National Survey on Drug Use and Health." September 2020. https://www.samhsa.gov/data/report/2019 -nsduh-annual-national-report.

———. "Locations Received Illicit Drug Use Treatment in Past Year among Persons Aged 12 or Older Who Received Illicit Drug Use Treatment at a Specialty Facility in Past Year by Percentages." Tables 5.25A and 5.25.B in "2019 NSDUH Detailed Tables." September 11, 2020. https://www.samhsa.gov/data/report/2019-nsduh-detailed-tables.

———. "Medications for Opioid Use Disorder: For Healthcare and Addiction Professionals, Policymakers, Patients, and Families." Treatment Improvement Protocol (TIP) Series 63. Last updated 2020. https://store.samhsa.gov/product/TIP-63-Medications-for-Opioid-Use-Disorder-Full-Document/PEP20-02-01-006.

———. "National Survey of Substance Abuse Treatment Services (N-SSATS): 2019 Data on Substance Abuse Treatment Services." Table 2.4. August 20, 2020. https://www.samhsa.gov/data/sites/default/files/reports/rpt29389/2019_NSSATS/2019_NSSATS_Tables.html#Tbl2.4.

———. "N-SSATS Facilities, by Status, Response Rate, Mode of Response, and State or Jurisdiction." Table 6.1 in "National Survey of Substance Abuse Treatment Services (N-SSATS): 2019 Data on Substance Abuse Treatment Facilities." August 20, 2020. https://www.samhsa.gov/data/sites/default/files/reports/rpt29389/2019_NSSATS/2019_NSSATS_Tables.html#Tbl6.1.

———. "An Overview of Treatment Improvement Protocol (TIP) 63: Medications for Opioid Use Disorder." February 1, 2018. https://www.samhsa.gov/sites/default/files/programs_campaigns/kap/tip-63_overview_of_treatment_ppt_7-11-18.pptx.

———. "Subtypes of Prescription Pain Relievers in the 2015 NSDUH Questionnaire." Figure 2 in "Prescription Drug Use and Misuse in the United States: Past Year Use of Subtypes of Prescription Drugs." *NSDUH Data Review*, September 2016. https://www.samhsa.gov/data/sites/default/files/NSDUH-FFR2-2015/NSDUH-FFR2-2015.htm#fig2.

———. "Subtypes of Prescription Sedatives in the 2015 NSDUH Questionnaire." Figure 5 in "Prescription Drug Use and Misuse in the United States: Past Year Use of Subtypes of Prescription Drugs." *NSDUH Data Review*, September 2016. https://www.samhsa.gov/data/sites/default/files/NSDUH-FFR2-2015/NSDUH-FFR2-2015.htm#fig5.

———. "Subtypes of Prescription Stimulants in the 2015 NSDUH Questionnaire." Figure 4 in "Prescription Drug Use and Misuse in the United States: Past Year Use of Subtypes of Prescription Drugs." *NSDUH Data Review*, September 2016. https://www.samhsa.gov/data/sites/default/files/NSDUH-FFR2-2015/NSDUH-FFR2-2015.htm#fig4.

———. "Subtypes of Prescription Tranquilizers in the 2015 NSDUH Questionnaire." Figure 3 in "Prescription Drug Use and Misuse in the United States: Past Year Use of Subtypes of Prescription Drugs." *NSDUH Data Review*, September 2016. https://www.samhsa.gov/data/sites/default/files/NSDUH-FFR2-2015/NSDUH-FFR2-2015.htm#fig3.

Tolbert, Jennifer, and Kendal Orgera. "Key Facts about the Uninsured Population." Kaiser Family Foundation, December 7, 2018. https://www.kff.org/uninsured/fact-sheet/key-facts-about-the-uninsured-population/.

Tolbert, Jennifer, Kendal Orgera, and Anthony Damico. "Key Facts about the Uninsured Population." Kaiser Family Foundation, November 6, 2020. https://www.kff.org/uninsured/issue-brief/key-facts-about-the-uninsured-population/.

US Government Spending. "What Is the Spending on Medicare?" January 4, 2021. https://www.usgovernmentspending.com/medicare_spending_by_year#:~:text=In%20FY%202020%20the%20federal,collections%2C%E2%80%9D%20was%20%24924%20billion.

Washington State Institute for Public Policy. "Benefit-Cost Results." Accessed May 26, 2021. http://www.wsipp.wa.gov/BenefitCost?topicId=7.

We Are Not Saints. https://wearenotsaints.com/.

Weber, Lauren. "How Political Maneuvering Derailed a Red State's Path to Medicaid Expansion." Kaiser Health News, September 6, 2019. https://khn.org/news/kansas-medicaid-expansion-conservative-political-playbook/.

Wen, Hefi, Jason M. Hockenberry, and Janet R. Cummings. "The Effect of Substance Use Disorder Treatment Use on Crime: Evidence from Public Insurance Expansions and Health Insurance Mandates." NBER Working Paper 20537. October 2014. https://www.nber.org/papers/w20537.pdf.

Zur, Julia, MaryBeth Musumeci, and Rachel Garfield. "Medicaid's Role in Financing Behavioral Health Services for Low-Income Individuals." Kaiser Family Foundation, June 29, 2017. https://www.kff.org/report-section/medicaids-role-in-financing-behavioral-health-services-for-low-income-individuals-issue-brief/.

INDEX

Page references for figures and tables are italicized.

ABOUT THE AUTHOR

Walter Wolf is a thirty-year veteran of the entertainment industry who produced studio and independent films and television throughout the United States, Australia, and South Africa. That all changed with one 3:00 a.m. call that a family member was in crisis due to addiction. Today, he is an interventionist helping families nationwide navigate the confusing world of addiction and mental illness treatment to find the right facility for their loved one. To know more about finding the right treatment for you or a loved one, go to therightrehab.com or call toll-free 1-855-702-7474 or email info@therightrehab.com.